Community Psychiatric Nursing

A Social Perspective

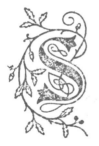

Community Psychiatric Nursing
A Social Perspective

Sue Simmons
Charlie Brooker

Heinemann Nursing
London

William Heinemann Medical Books
22 Bedford Square
London WC1B 3HH

ISBN 0–433–30290–9

First published 1986
Reprinted 1987

Typeset by Latimer Trend & Company Ltd, Plymouth
Printed and bound in Great Britain by
Biddles Ltd, Guildford and King's Lynn

Contents

Dedication

To our partners – Roger and Linda who have given us endless support and encouragement

Acknowledgements

It is impossible to thank directly all the people who have contributed to the ideas in this book, including of course all the members of Bloomsbury CPN service, who have demonstrated that ideas and developments often arise out of the commitment, energy and hard work of a team. However, a number of people have made some very particular contributions. A large group has read and made helpful comments on earlier drafts of particular chapters, including Rosemary Wadsworth, Emma Fayter, Dennis Parrish, Helen Lee, Moira Coombes, Ted White, Lis Jones, Mick Hunt and Cathy Watson. In addition Roger Croot read and commented in some detail on many of the chapters. Our thanks go to all for their time and interest.

We would also like to thank Paul Beard and Christine Hancock, who as senior nurse managers created a milieu within Bloomsbury Health Authority in which new ideas, practices and innovations were fostered.

We are grateful to the Community Psychiatric Nurses Association for permission to quote most of the factual information in Chapter 3, and to Jen Waterton for her expert statistical advice in this area.

Finally, our thanks to Chris Botterill who typed Chapters 3 and 7.

Foreword

This book is to be welcomed as a contribution to the debate on how community nursing can develop alternative methods of mental health care in the place where the patient lives. As it explains, the medical model of mental illness is only one approach to mental distress. There are other approaches which may tackle more effectively the very important issues of bad environments, interfamily problems and the social pressures of everyday life.

Society is in the midst of major change, and mental health services are no exception. Nurse education must reflect the need for collaboration with social services and housing agencies, as well as with the carers of people with mental health problems who live at home or with relatives. Community nurses are in an excellent position to develop keyworker approaches to the needs of those requiring long-term support in the community and to offer a channel for the provision of resources to people in their own homes. Through it, nursing will be revalued as a profession—which can only be to the good, as long as nurses recognise the other important specialities with which they should work, and the need to develop generic care staff who can provide the regular day-to-day contact with those who have long-term and continuing disabilities.

This is a singularly appropriate moment in which to publish a new book on community psychiatric nursing. Although full-fledged community care may still be some way off, the development of alternatives to institutions is accelerating. Suddenly we are seeing health authority plans for community care come to some sort of fruition. This transition is very positive, but it constitutes a major upheaval which is causing discomfort to the management and staff of the institutions, to the patients who have not been properly prepared, and to a community suspicious about the arrival of mental health care in its midst.

In all of this the community psychiatric nurse is one of the key professionals. The CPN's value is that of a well-qualified professional with "hands on" experience, yet without a vested interest in preserving the narrow institutional approach to mental illness. CPNs are in a good position to take direct referrals from general practitioners, to link with GP clinics to undertake counselling and preventive work, and to work with schools and colleges. Many community nurses are drawn from black and ethnic minority groups and will therefore be in a good position to ensure that those communities get the services that they need.

Getting nurses out of the institutions and into the community was a farsighted move which has helped to bridge the gap between community and hospital—acting as a bridge in both ways—enabling a sensitive and well-supported move for many patients to a more fulfilled life in the community, while continuing to support the patients on an outreach basis. On the other hand, there is a danger which is all too evident. CPNs could be seen to be the institution *in* the community, preserving the medical domination of mental health services and the institutionalising effects of that approach.

Community psychiatric nursing is one of the success stories of the mental health services over the last thirty years. The development of community care needs a staff-intensive service which can operate locally and accessibly, delivering care wherever possible *to* the patient. Because of the past lack of proper planning for the development of alternatives to institutions, giving staff an exciting and viable future is an important step towards developing the care that is needed. Positive approaches to community psychiatric nursing such as this book provides will encourage hesitant staff that there is a future outside of institutions. The chill wind that many fear blows outside the institutional walls is clearly not so chill after all.

Christopher J. Heginbotham
National Director
MIND

Preface

It is our intention and hope that this book will be relevant to those currently working as community psychiatric nurses, registered mental nurse students on CPN placements, those working in other community mental health services, whether nurses or other professionals, and anyone else interested in this challenging field.

Although this has been a joint project by the two authors, the main responsibility for chapters is as follows:

Sue Simmons: Chapters 1, 2, 4, 5 and 6.
Charlie Brooker: Chapters 3 and 7

Sue Simmons is Lecturer in Community Psychiatric Nursing at North East London Polytechnic. She was formerly Assistant Director of Nursing Services (Community Mental Health), Bloomsbury Health Authority.

Charlie Brooker is Senior Lecturer in Community Psychiatric Nursing at Sheffield Polytechnic. He was formerly Senior Nurse (Research and Planning), Bloomsbury Health Authority.

1
Introduction

Community psychiatric nursing and mental health services in general are now, for many different reasons, at a critical point in their history. There have been far-reaching changes in the treatment of and attitudes towards those suffering from mental illness over the past decades, and the pattern of mental health services is now changing markedly in many countries. The many current developments in community psychiatric nursing are taking place against this background. We shall mention here some of the features of these changes, and the main issues now facing psychiatric nursing in the community, many of which will be discussed more fully in later chapters.

It is impossible to refer to the very practical changes that have occurred in mental health services without also considering the changes in attitude and ideology that have accompanied them. During the last century the Victorians built numerous very large psychiatric asylums, often in pleasant country settings geographically isolated from residential areas. Within these, many thousands of patients lived, often for all of their adult lives, sometimes losing all contact with their family, friends and the outside world. Although the motives of those who established these institutions may well have been humanitarian (to provide people with space, fresh air and an accepting environment), the asylums also served the function of removing people with disturbed and distressing behaviour from mainstream society. The general public seldom had to become involved or attempt to understand the problem. We now know that such custodial care greatly exacerbated the problems of the people who were admitted – by fostering passivity and dependence, by reinforcing unusual behaviour and by destroying their sense of identity.

During this century there have been many changes, some of

which have been fairly radical. In the field of treatment there have been developments in new forms of chemotherapy, in particular the neuroleptics, and growing expertise among mental health professionals in non-drug therapies, including counselling, behaviour therapy, family therapy, social skills training and so on. There is now greater awareness of the damaging effects of institutional care. As a result, the range of possible settings for the delivery of care has become much wider. In the past treatment was carried out in hospital or the out-patient department. Now it may be provided in an almost infinite variety of locations, including day hospital, day centre, health centre, social services department, general practitioner surgery, mental health centre – and of course people's homes.

Some mental health professionals have also been influenced by the anti-psychiatry movement which has questioned many of the fundamental assumptions about mental illness. Among professionals and lay people there has been an increased interest in the part played by the family and society in creating or exacerbating ill-health. Linked to these changes, and in parallel to them, there has been some change in society's attitude towards those with mental ill-health. Mental illness and psychological problems can now be discussed in a way that would have been almost unthinkable in the not-so-distant past. There are now frequent television documentaries, plays and newspaper articles on schizophrenia, phobias, anorexia nervosa and depression. Although such media coverage does not necessarily allay fears or increase understanding (although it can do), it has lead to the acknowledgement of the existence and problems of mental ill-health. We could say that mental illness has at last come out of the closet!

This is not to suggest that there is no longer any misunderstanding or fear about mental ill-health or that there is now no stigma attached to those who receive psychiatric treatment. Sadly, this is very far from the case as many community psychiatric nurses will know. For example, we are all aware of the potential difficulty of setting up a new group-home in a residential area where the neighbours might well protest and prevent the plans proceeding. But the recent moves to develop much more community care, and to resettle long-stay hospital patients into homes within the community, will at least now be familiar to many members of the general public, even if the policy is not supported by them.

There has, then, been a major shift in thinking away from providing treatment in large institutions towards the provision of local home-based care for as many people as possible. Such care is not only much more therapeutic, but it also prevents the individual developing many of the handicaps that can be brought about by an institutional stay. When someone is admitted to in-patient care, he or she will generally have to relinquish or modify many of the roles he or she plays on a day-to-day basis, for example: employee, work colleague, neighbour, parent, church member, etc. Even otherwise able and confident people may feel overawed by the hospital system. In contrast, by providing care and treatment in people's home environments, we do not put them in the position of having to give up all of these. Rather, certain parts of their lives will usually remain untouched by their mental health problem, self-esteem is less threatened, treatment is less disruptive to themselves and their families, and the stigma of having a psychiatric problem is reduced. As a result, therapy can aim to mobilise an individual's strengths and to be the minimum necessary to restore the person to his or her previous life pattern.

Many supporters of developments in community care do recognise, however, the definite need for some in-patient provision in the future, whatever facilities exist in the community. There will almost certainly be a need for asylum for those in acute breakdown and a secure environment for those who could otherwise be a threat to themselves or others.

But what do we mean by "community" and – perhaps more importantly – "community care"? There have been various efforts to define these terms, which are both rather ambiguous, in recent years. A community can be a particular district, a local neighbourhood, a segment of a larger society or a way of life (as in an ethnic community). A report by the Richmond Fellowship (1983) suggests that community may refer to a geographically-defined district for which certain authorities have responsibilities or a well-integrated neighbourhood where people know each other and nobody is isolated.

Similarly, community care may be thought of as care *in* the community, or care *by* the community. Again there are certainly differing views – particularly between, on the one hand, some of the professionals providing community services who tend to think in terms of the former and, on the other hand, some politicians who determine policy and tend to favour the latter. Some of the voluntary organisations in the mental health field would also like to see care by the community developed. For example, the Richmond Fellowship argues that community care should, first, refer to the responsibilities of the health and local authorities for a particular district but that, second, a part of these responsibilities is to encourage the well-integrated neighbourhood that they describe. There are also differing views about the financial implications of the proposals of many Regional Health Authorities to close down their large psychiatric hospitals in the next five or ten years. This is sometimes interpreted as a cost-cutting exercise, although many people now think that the development of a local comprehensive mental health service will cost as much as, if not more than, the old institutions.

Community Psychiatric Nursing – Looking Forward

There has been a great deal of movement in recent decades, but there is still a long way to go towards the type of mental health service that many people would like to see. But what is the situation for community psychiatric nurses (CPNs)?

In the relatively short period of time since the first community psychiatric nursing services were established, there has been great expansion, both in new teams being set up and further posts being established within existing services. For many years the setting-up of new CPN services, whether done slowly or more rapidly, has been virtually ignored by those who did not have day-to-day contact with mental health services. This has allowed a certain amount of *ad hoc* development and an opportunity for CPNs to build up skills, knowledge and some sense of professional identity. In some areas the opportunity has been seized with enthusiasm and CPN services have thrived, while in other areas resources have been scarcer and CPNs have been few in number. However, the days of *ad hoc* and patchy growth may soon be past. Several recent government reports have included recommendations on the work and training of CPNs, there is talk of regional guidelines on staffing levels, and in many districts there is now an expectation that CPN services should systematically describe and evaluate their work.

Several issues that face CPNs and those who manage them are now being discussed both within and outside the profession. Despite the growth in the number of CPNs over the past two decades the total is still fairly small (approximately 3500 in 1985). There are now additional plans for massive further expansion in

CPN numbers. Further growth will require greater clarity and agreement about the path that services should take.

CPNs could move along two main paths in the future. The first would be to become more involved in primary health care, health education and the prevention of mental ill-health. This is already happening in many districts where CPNs may be attached to or based in local health centres, accepting referrals from all staff who work there. Such a move away from the traditional psychiatric hospital base would increase the number of clients referred and dramatically widen the range of problems of the clients seen. The second main direction would be for CPN services to take a particularly active part in the setting up of community care for the residents of psychiatric hospitals, many of whom have been in hospital for a large part of their adult lives. This role has been advocated by the director of the Health Advisory Service, and endorsed by the Social Services Select Committee (1985): "The CPN is probably the most important single professional in the process of moving care of mental illness into the community".

These two aspects of a CPN's role may appear divergent and incompatible, but it is best to see them as complementary. Neither should be sacrificed in order to concentrate on the other, and both should be seen as the legitimate business of a CPN service. This is not to say that individual CPNs would or should be able to take on all the many new areas of work, but that the service as a whole should see itself as having a responsibility for clients with a wide range of mental health problems.

In addition to the issues within the profession, there are also discussions about the relationships between CPNs and other disciplines, in particular the other professions in the mental health field, including psychiatrists, psychologists, occupational therapists, and social workers. In many districts, teams of different workers, with CPNs as core members, are being set up to provide a community mental health service. CPNs in such districts are no longer working semi-autonomously within a nursing team, but as key-workers within a multidisciplinary team. In such teams there is inevitably a blurring of professional boundaries, and the overlap of roles that already exists is further enlarged. Perhaps to reflect this role-overlap, a rather different proposal has been put forward by MIND in their manifesto *Common Concern* (MIND, 1983). This document suggests a new staff group called community mental health workers. The training of these generic workers would combine elements of the training of social workers, occupational therapists, community psychiatric nurses and other care workers. Community mental health workers would provide the service previously provided by these separate disciplines.

Another debate in which CPNs are involved concerns the future educational requirements of psychiatric nurses in general and CPNs in particular, at a time when nurse education as a whole is under scrutiny.

In view of all these developments and debates, now is a time of great opportunity and potential confusion for CPNs. There is an increasing need for a consensus about the nature, scope and future direction of community psychiatric nursing, primarily within the profession itself, but also among the many other disciplines and organisations with whom CPNs work. We do not suggest that there should be standardisation or uniformity among CPN services, but that there is a need for a framework within which CPN services and individual CPNs may work.

The development of such a consensus is not easy. We shall not attempt at this stage to define what a CPN is, or what the role and functions of CPNs are, since it is our view that there are no simple answers to these questions. Rather, we intend that the following chapters will draw the outline and paint in some of the details. For the present it is worth noting that CPN services have developed in many different ways, and that this is indeed one of their strengths. Some teams have been set up from the beginning within primary health care services. More commonly, teams have been established as part of the overall mental health services, often initially to take on out-patient and follow-up work. Within both types of services, any further expansion has happened in parallel with more general moves to provide more care in the community.

But how do CPNs see their role and the meaning of community care? In her research on a CPN service in Edinburgh, Sladden (1979) attempted to discover how CPNs interpreted community care. She found that they did this in three main ways, all of which suggest concepts of care in the community:

- care by social agencies, as opposed to hospital services
- any care given without admission to hospital
- a comprehensive system of preventive psychiatry, including a range of services.

The nurses appeared to adopt different definitions depending on their working environment. From a hospital base the CPN tended to use the first model which clearly separates medical and social care. From a community base there was greater identification with the needs of the client and family and less demarcation of the CPNs' work. Although the nurses used all three models in different settings, Sladden found that they aspired to the third model as the ideal.

We also see community care as requiring a comprehensive system of services, underpinned by a number of principles, including: a recognition of a person's right to receive treatment and care in the home environment wherever possible; to receive the best possible care, based on individual needs, and endeavouring to promote self-determination and minimise dependence; to maintain his or her right to make choices; and to remain integrated with the rest of society. Such care will prevent many people from developing a more serious mental health problem, and for others will reduce the level of the handicaps they suffer as a result of ill-health.

If the word "community" in the title "community psychiatric nurse" is ambiguous, the word "psychiatric" can be quite contentious! Part of the diversity among CPN services and the wish for self-determination has led some nurses to use different ways of describing themselves (for example, community mental health nurse, mental health practitioner, etc.). This probably reflects a changing perspective on the work being carried out and a desire to loosen the links with what is seen as traditional psychiatry. We have used the term community psychiatric nurse throughout this book, not because we see this title as necessarily the most appropriate, but because it is at present the most widespread and well-known. We have also used this title because we think that CPN services should strive to maintain a balance between developing new ventures which could potentially widen the range of people making use of them, and providing a community nursing service to those who have had a generally acknowledged and probably major psychiatric illness. We do, however, use the term "client" rather than "patient" for those who receive the care of CPNs. This is now commonly used in many districts. It reflects the more equal relationship between the providers and the users of CPN services, where much of the care and treatment is provided away from the nurse's base and often in the client's home.

Outline of the Book

Our perspective on mental health is psychosocial. We see people not as totally separate entities, divorced from the rest of society, but as influencing and being influenced by it. We will attempt to place the individual firmly within the context of his or her family, the community and the wider society, and to show that interaction occurs at all these levels. We will introduce the concept of systems, in order to consider the individual client as a member of a family system or community, and also to examine the world and the work of the CPN as a member of several professional systems. Although we will be quite open about our own views on the nature of community psychiatric nursing and the direction it should take, we attempt to represent and discuss fairly the wide range of services, organisations and approaches that exist. As far as possible we use findings from research studies within nursing and related disciplines, as we hope to encourage a questioning and investigative approach to practice.

In Chapter 2 we introduce some theory and research from different disciplines, including sociology, that have contributed to philosophies of care, and that provide us with a wider perspective from which to examine community mental health issues. We include some of the social factors that appear to affect the distribution or reporting of mental ill-health, and some of the demographic changes occurring in our society. This chapter ends with an examination of some of the mental health and social policies that provide the background to the development of CPN services.

In Chapter 3 we discuss the development, structure and organisation of CPN services, using as our basis the 1980 and 1985 CPNA surveys. CPN services vary in many different ways, including the bases from which team members work, their referral systems, the numbers and grading of staff within a service, their training, and the degree of specialisation. This chapter concludes by drawing together geographical, structural and philosophical factors which combine to affect the overall aims of CPN services.

We turn to considering the CPN client in Chapter 4, and look at the environment and system surrounding a person, in particular his or her immediate family. We begin by discussing what is meant by a "family system" and refer to the normal patterns of cycles and events for individuals and families. We consider the work of the CPN in terms of assessment, the planning of care, and interventions. The chapter includes a discussion of clients requiring long-term care, including those who may be moving back into the community after a long hospitalisation, as well as those who have short-term or medium-term needs. As the role of families in the provision of care is important and increasingly so, we consider some aspects of family burden, family atmosphere and the family carers' needs for support.

In Chapter 5 we consider the individual as a member of a wider system, by which we mean their neighbourhood and society at large. We discuss community and social factors that appear to affect mental health, for example community integration, unemployment and housing. We shall also consider the CPN's role in working with groups of people, whether they be groups focused specifically on mental health issues or those established for a different purpose. The theme of health education and preventive work arises in several parts of the book, including a section of this chapter (p. 114). We also briefly consider the current discussions about the nurse's role as the patient/client's advocate, and finish with a short section on some aspects of housing policy, welfare benefits and occupational opportunities pertinent to people with mental health problems.

Chapter 6 concentrates on the community psychiatric nurse, by considering his or her environment, work situation and surrounding systems. This includes: the CPN's team organisation; need for support; supervision; key relationships with primary health care services; psychiatric services; nursing colleagues; social services and voluntary agencies; and data collection. In a section on the political arena, we discuss the bodies with statutory powers within nursing, and the various organisations representing the interests of community psychiatric nursing in particular. We also consider the potential political role of community nurses.

In our final chapter (7) we turn to the future and comment on some of the most important and sometimes controversial issues now facing community psychiatric nursing. We discuss four main topics:

- The future education of CPNs, acknowledging the moves towards mandatory training.
- The role of research in the development of community psychiatric nursing.
- The debate on specialism and generalism.

● Where does community psychiatric nursing go from here?

Many readers will prefer to start with particular chapters rather than read the book from start to finish. There are, however, references to different chapters at several points, and the themes already mentioned will run throughout the book. We hope that it will be stimulating and occasionally provocative. In addition, we hope that it will contribute to the continuing debate about psychiatric nursing in the community.

References

MIND (1983) *Common Concern*. MIND Publications, London.
Richmond Fellowship (1983) *Mental Health and the Community*. Richmond Fellowship, London.
Sladden, S. (1979) *Psychiatric Nursing in the Community*. Churchill Livingstone, Edinburgh.
Social Services Select Committee (1985) *Community Care*, Vol 1. HMSO, London.

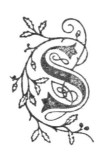

2
Setting the Scene

The definition of what constitutes mental illness is beset with problems. The number of people seeking psychiatric care, whether as in-patients or out-patients, has been estimated at 600 000 per year, with a further 5 million consulting their general practitioner each year with some mental health problem (Ineichen, 1979). Such straightforward counting of patients and clients implies that the issues are simple when, in fact, they are not. For example, the supply of psychiatric services influences the demand (the more beds available, the greater the bed occupancy; the more CPNs there are and the better they are known, the more referrals to the service), and there are many additional factors that need to be taken into consideration when attempts to define psychiatric illness or count psychiatric patients are made.

The most common model of psychiatric illness used in the hospital setting is the medical model. Many nurses working in the community have moved away from using this model to account for the problems that beset their clients, and indeed we find several drawbacks if we apply it to people with mental health problems. Cochrane (1983) outlines three limitations:

- The medical model requires some notion of "normal" mental health.
- The quest for a definitive diagnosis can divert the professional's attention away from helping the person with the problems that she or he faces.
- The model almost inevitably leads to an emphasis on physical forms of treatment without great knowledge of how these treatments work.

There are several reasons for these limitations to the medical model.

(1) CPNs quickly discover that normal mental health must be individually defined, and that family, social and cultural factors must be considered. As Cochrane suggests, one of the reasons that psychiatry may fail to "cure" is that it often continues to ignore the social context of a person's problems and treats him or her in isolation. The ideas that a person has about health and illness are influenced by his family and subculture, so there is wide variation in what is considered good health (for a full discussion on this see Clare, 1976).

(2) It also becomes evident to CPNs that clients and their families are more concerned with the behavioural, interpersonal and psychological manifestations of their mental health problems than with any psychiatric diagnoses. For example, the effects of a woman's depression on family relationships and her husband's performance at work are more pressing issues to her and her family than her precise diagnosis.

(3) Medication and other physical treatments may provide temporary relief, and in some cases long-term stability, but they are not the answer in all cases, particularly where there may be multiple problems.

There is a fourth disadvantage to the medical model when applied to mental health. The medical profession in western culture has a commitment to intervention in what it defines as illness (Dingwall, 1976). Within psychological medicine this can lead to a seeking out of illness where previously problems were conceptualised as social, cultural or even moral. In addition, just as those suffering from psychological distress variably define mental ill-health, so too do doctors. Ineichen (1979) refers to reports on the percentage of GP consultations which are for mental health problems as estimated by the GPs involved. The majority of GPs estimated that around 12–14% of their consultations were for mental health problems, but among the other GPs the highest estimates were between eight and nine times higher than the lowest, indicating a very wide range. Some of this range may be accounted for by the characteristics of the population of a particular area, but it is likely that the doctor's interest in, and therefore predisposition to seek out, psychological problems will play a major part. In this case the general practitioners could be said to be determining the reported extent of mental illness. Similarly, two or more psychiatrists from different backgrounds may not diagnose the same condition in the same person; that is, there may be a low level of replicability of diagnosis. For example, in the United States psychiatrists are more likely to diagnose schizophrenia in "borderline" cases than are psychiatrists in the United Kingdom (Cooper *et al.*, 1972).

A further criticism of the medical model has come from labelling theorists who have argued that the use of a diagnosis causes otherwise sporadic behaviour to become a regular feature for the labelled individual.

If, then, we move away from wholesale use of concepts like diagnosis and prognosis which are drawn from medicine (although at times they may still be of value), what do we put in their place? We suggest that an eclectic approach is required and is better than simply adopting one simple model to explain and address all the multitude of mental health problems that may be found in our society. This approach can be built up by considering some of the work that has been done in the field of mental health and mental illness by social scientists from other disciplines.

Sociology and Mental Illness

What is labelling?

The term "labelling" has come to be used fairly widely within psychiatric circles and, generally speaking, one of the aims of the move towards community care is to reduce the likelihood of labelling occurring and to lessen its damaging impact when it does happen.

The term originated in the sociology of deviance where mental illness was studied as an example of deviant behaviour. The labelling theory of deviance claims that: "social groups create deviance by making the rules whose infraction constitutes deviance, and by applying those rules to particular people and labelling them as outsiders" (Becker, 1963, p. 9). According to this theory, whether certain rule-breaking behaviour is labelled as deviant will depend on the reaction of society, rather than solely on the nature of the behaviour itself.

Scheff (1966) has related some of these ideas to the field of mental illness. (It is important to bear in mind that almost all the work in this area concentrates on psychotic illnesses, in particular schizophrenic disorders.) He adopts the term "residual rule-breaking" to refer to diverse kinds of behaviour that cannot easily be categorised as another form of deviance, including withdrawal, hallucinations and posturing. In certain situations these behaviours would be quite appropriate, for example, in a meditation session or a seance, but if seen in a public setting they are viewed as odd and unacceptable. Such behaviour has also been described as "primary" deviance – that is, deviant behaviour before it is officially labelled.

Frequently those close to the person displaying this behaviour will seek alternative explanations: for example, that the person has been working too hard and is in need of a rest, that he is physically ill, affected by drugs or fatigued. In many situations, especially if the behaviour is temporary, this form of accounting will be successful. Other factors, called contingencies, may affect whether the residual rule-breaker will move further in the direction of being given a label of mental illness (Goffman, 1961). These include the nature of the rule-breaking, and its seriousness and visibility; the influence and position in society of the person who breaks the rules; the tolerance level of the community; and the person's relationships with key people, including his or her family.

In other words, and to simplify the argument, an episode of withdrawal and odd inexplicable behaviour may be viewed, responded to, and hence labelled very differently if the individual is a middle-aged family man who has been working very hard in a demanding job, than if he is a young itinerant with no regular employment or accommodation.

Scheff calls the process by which alternative explanations are sought "denial", and argues that most residual rule-breaking is denied. Various studies have investigated the prevalence of psychological problems in the community, and most have found that there are far higher rates than one would expect from looking at the people who reach the psychiatric services (see, for example, Brown and Harris, 1978). Community surveys report having found psychiatric symptoms in as many as a quarter or a half of the sample, depending on the criteria used (Ineichen, 1979). Clearly, some of these people may be treated by their general practitioners, but a large proportion will remain undetected and may not define themselves as having a mental health problem. Some writers suggest that virtually all of us experience what could be defined as symptoms of psychiatric illness at different times in our lives, for example, depression or excessive anxiety.

If, however, denial does not occur and doubts are raised so that others begin to respond to the person as if he were possibly mentally ill, the odd behaviour is reinforced and withdrawal becomes greater. A vicious circle develops. Gradually the individual himself begins to adopt the label that has been applied and to behave accordingly. This response of the individual to society's reaction is called "secondary" deviance, and it is this deviant behaviour for which, it is claimed, society is partly responsible. Labelling theorists suggest that when professionals describe a patient as developing "insight" into his illness they are, in effect, rewarding his acceptance of the deviant mentally ill role. If an individual adopts an alternative explanation for his behaviour, this may be met by disapproval. For example, Laing (1976a) quotes a discussion between a "catatonic schizophrenic" and his therapist:

> *Patient*   When I came back from Vietnam, it was too confus-
> ing, too complex. I had to try to figure it out .... So I
> finally made no movements at all. They carted me here. I
> realised that I couldn't simplify my life this way, so I
> started to move normally again, and talk....
> *Therapist*   But John, I thought you were really cured and now
> I hear that you have been putting on a show to get out. I
> am disappointed in you.

Once a label is assigned, previous behaviour is assessed retro-spectively and often incorporated into the new theory. Goffman (1961) cites the use of case-notes in a mental hospital as being records of all past incidents in the person's life and family history that have significance with regard to the person's diagnosis, rather than as an average sample of previous experiences.

This last finding was experienced by some researchers in the USA who got themselves admitted to different psychiatric hospi-tals by complaining of hearing voices saying "empty", "thud" and "hollow" (Rosenhan, 1979). All but one were diagnosed as schizophrenic and all were undetected by staff (although not always by fellow patients!). It was some time before any of them were discharged as schizophrenics in remission, despite the fact that they stopped their complaints of hallucinations as soon as they were admitted and told staff that they felt completely well. They found (as Goffman had done) that the staff's interpretation of their life histories and current behaviour (for example, their writing up of research notes on the ward) was shaped to fit their diagnoses.

> Nursing records for three patients indicate that the writing was seen as an aspect of their pathological behaviour. "Patient engages in writing behaviour" was the daily nursing comment on one of the pseudopatients who was never questioned about his writing (Rosenhan, 1979, p. 91).

Throughout their admission the pseudopatients behaved as they would have done normally and answered questions about their backgrounds honestly.

One of the conclusions of this study was that any diagnostic exercise which leads to such major errors cannot be very reliable. However, Clare (1976) has argued convincingly that the results highlight the need for the diagnostic process to be very thorough, careful and based on more than one symptom, rather than that the attempt should be abandoned completely.

Earlier we referred also to the tendency of medicine to adopt an interventionist approach and to seek out illness where it may not be immediately apparent. Rosenhan's experiment appears to provide some demonstration of this tendency.

Similarly, Scheff in his research found that doctors, when in doubt, will err on the side of diagnosing sickness in someone who is well, rather than health in someone who is ill. He argues that in general medicine an incorrect diagnosis of illness, when in fact the patient is healthy, will do little or no long-term harm. (We would agree, provided that the incorrect diagnosis does not lead to highly intrusive treatment such as surgery!) However, Scheff argues, this absence of harm may not be the case in the field of psychiatry, where there is still unfortunately often a stigma attached to a psychiatric label.

The value of labelling theory

We have discussed labelling theory, at some length, not because we wish to adopt it in its entirety (any more than we would wish to adopt the medical model of psychiatric illness completely), but because we think it has something important to say to those working in community mental health and psychiatric services generally. One young woman, writing about her experiences in hospital when she had a schizophrenic breakdown, describes the power of the expectations of others better than we can (Horne, 1985, p. 35). She remembers two general student nurses as particularly helpful for a somewhat surprising reason:

> The next (thing they did) was to sit down with my friend and me to chat – as though we were four office clerks in our coffee break . . . . It was difficult to give in to symptoms when these two nurses were around. It was easy to behave schizophrenically when someone expected it . . . . But I could not possibly embarrass myself in front of two people who only ever saw me as being just like themselves. Since I could not give in to symptoms they and everyone else saw me as normal and I behaved more sanely and felt more mentally stable.

In its purest form labelling theory (and perhaps the above quote) would appear to argue that mental illness (in fact psychotic mental illness) does not exist apart from where it has been defined by those with the authority to label, that it is a construct created by society, and that mentally ill people are simply those so defined. On the face of it this appears to be a cold denial of the pain and suffering felt by individuals and their families, with which nurses working in the community will be only too familiar. Interestingly, however, neither Scheff nor Rosenhan are arguing such a case. Scheff says that he has deliberately put forward an argument opposed to that of the generally accepted individual system model (for example, the medical, psychoanalytical or behavioural models) in order to highlight the importance of social and cultural factors in the processes surrounding someone becoming mentally ill. He admits that he has almost certainly exaggerated the importance of these, but says that this has been necessary in order to make a case for an eventual synthesis of the two perspectives.

The value of labelling theory to community psychiatric nurses is that it gives us insights into the many different processes that may play a part in the lives and experiences of people referred to our CPN services. This is the case despite the fact that Scheff's work focuses only on those with chronic mental illness. By being familiar with the sociological perspective we will be more able to recognise the important part played by the context of someone's behaviour. In addition to the relatively static social variables that appear to play their part in influencing psychological problems, we can now add:

- The interactive process between the person and significant others.
- The reaction of the wider society, often affected by the person's status, the degree of oddness in his behaviour, and the availability of alternative explanations.
- The willingness, or otherwise, of the person to accept others' definitions of what is happening.

It is, of course, possible that the mental health services, including the CPN, could play a part in affecting the course of psychological disturbance. The mental health services generally are becoming more accessible; hence people who may not in the past have thought of themselves as being in need of such help may now be seeing a psychiatrist or psychiatric nurse for counselling. Is it possible that what would have previously been described as "life problems" (to do with housing, employment, normal reactions to stressful events, etc.) are now being seen as mental health problems, to the potential disadvantage of the client? We think that the mental health service should be more accessible and indeed we put the case for increasing the mental health input at primary care level in a later chapter, but we are simply raising this as a potential dilemma.

Role and status

The second theme from sociology that we want to consider in relation to mental health involves the concepts of status and role. These concepts are also important in social psychology. Everyone within a society occupies a number of positions or statuses. Some of these are fixed or ascribed – for example, one's sex and, in some societies, caste. Although it is not fixed, we could also consider age as an ascribed status, since it is not alterable. Other statuses are achieved, perhaps through some purposive action by the status-holder – for example, one's occupation or marital status.

Statuses are accompanied by a set of "norms" which define, more or less rigidly, the rights, expectations and obligations of the individual occupying a particular status. These norms make up the "role".

It is helpful to think of three types of roles (Banton, 1965):

Basic roles, which are predetermined and therefore correspond to the ascribed statuses of sex, age, ethnic group, etc.; they are described as basic since they define how an individual is expected to behave and how others respond to him in a wide variety of settings.

General roles, which are less far-reaching, but still bring with them restrictions and privileges, and which tend to affect other areas of the person's life: for example, the roles attached to the statuses of prisoner or parent, or to some occupational statuses like doctor, sailor or priest.

Independent roles, with fewer implications and probably little or no influence on other roles, for example most occupations, hobbies, etc.

The taking on of roles is first learned in childhood within the family, at school and in peer groups, but is then continued in life through the process of socialisation. An individual will hold many different roles and will move from one to another many times during the course of a day. Some roles will be complementary to the roles of others, for example, customer and shop-assistant, nurse and patient. When different roles held by one person are not compatible, he or she will experience role-strain or role-conflict.

The degree to which a role carries explicit instructions of expected behaviour, type of dress and so on is variable. Some writers believe that most roles provide guidelines only and are often unclear and ambiguous. The participants in a situation therefore negotiate, clarify and improvise to reach agreement. It is possible to view illness, including mental illness, in this way by considering what has been called the "sick role". Just as other roles imply a number of rights and responsibilities, so too does the sick role. The person is seen to have a responsibility to seek out appropriate help and to take the advice he is given. He should see being ill as undesirable and want to get well. In return he is relieved by others of many of his responsibilities, for example, his work and tasks at home.

How then does the status of sick person with its accompanying role come about? In many situations a status and its role are both arrived at together – for example, when a person takes on a new job. In physical illness a person may seek help, and hence take on the sick role, when he is unable to reconcile his symptoms with his everyday life. This need not be at the point of maximum severity. The idea that someone is sick may be socially determined by various factors, only one of which is the actual biological disease present (Mangen, 1982). Dingwall (1976, p. 59) points out that "'Illnesses' are terms employed by sufferers, and those with whom they interact, to make sense of events in their lives". The process of adopting the sick role may be extended over time.

This may happen even more commonly in the case of mental ill-health, where what could be considered symptomatic behaviour may be displayed by the individual possibly for some time before the status of ill person is used by himself or others. There is evidence, as we mentioned earlier, that signs of psychological problems are frequently undetected for some time, and that they may be deliberately overlooked or denied by family and friends. The status of sick person is, it seems, negotiated over time. Initially, and especially if the problem is thought to be short-term, it is likely that the sick role will be "independent" – that is, it will not have many consequences for other roles. However, if the problem becomes longer-term, or if the person is perhaps admitted to psychiatric hospital, it will become a "general" role with far-reaching effects. The label of mentally ill person has been described as a "master status" which affects all other statuses that the person holds. In the case of mental illness, far more than in the case of physical illness, the change in people's roles and statuses will affect how others will react to them and how they view themselves. Many CPNs will be able to recall countless examples of such changes in role being experienced by their clients.

There is another way in which mental illness appears to differ from most physical illness, and that is in how it is thought of by others. "'Illness' is only understandable and meaningful to people if it is in contradistinction to normal 'health'" (Robinson, 1971). Being ill is generally considered to be temporary. Therefore, if someone has what appears to be a long-term – perhaps permanent – mental illness, Robinson suggests that this may be reinterpreted as their normal state, and another status is assigned. Such a status change may, of course, also apply to those with permanent physical disabilities.

Social Factors in Mental Health

We have been discussing social processes which over the course of time would appear to have an effect on mental health or illness. It is also possible to identify certain social factors which have been linked to mental health problems.

Each individual is, of course, unique. No amount of unravelling of the social and environmental factors that may affect mental health will fully account for the personal and interpersonal complexity of one individual and his or her family. Every day CPNs meet clients who do not fit into the expected pattern. Nevertheless, by being familiar with some of the variables that have been shown to be correlated with higher levels of reported mental ill-health, nurses working in the community may be able to increase their understanding of the problems facing their clients. This will help them to plan good nursing care more effectively.

Such knowledge is also particularly useful when we look beyond the caseload of an individual CPN and consider how best to meet the mental health needs of the population of a district or "patch". This requires us to take into account how the population of that area is constituted. What is the male/female ratio? What age-groups are disproportionately large or small? Is it predominantly established residential or a mixed area with a rapid population turnover? What types of housing exist? Are the levels of unemployment high? The answers to such questions are of fundamental interest to individual CPNs and their teams in getting to know their particular area, and are not simply the province of the planners and service managers. The following section therefore gives a brief overview of the main factors that have been identified as being linked to mental health and illness.

Sex differences

Perhaps the most striking observation that has been made over and over again is the different proportions of males and females who are admitted to psychiatric hospitals, attend out-patients or are on CPN caseloads. One woman in eight as compared to one man in twelve will be admitted to in-patient psychiatric care at some point in their lives (MIND, 1980). Within in-patient populations, men with schizophrenic diagnoses outnumber such women, but women outnumber men in depression and other neurotic conditions. Male suicides also outnumber those of women, although the positions are reversed for self-injury. Not surprisingly in view of the differences in diagnoses, the peak age for men being admitted is the early 20s, while for women it is middle-age, with an additional earlier peak of women in their late 20s consulting their general practitioners with mental health problems (Mangen, 1982).

The overall gender difference in utilisation of mental health services may be related in some way to another consistent difference between men and women. Surveys in the UK and USA show that women generally report more ill-health in themselves than do men, and women use medical services more (Nathanson, 1978). Yet despite women's apparently greater morbidity, men have a higher mortality rate and as a result a shorter life expectancy. Three main models have been put forward to explain these differences.

(1) The differences reflect different levels of "real" illness between the sexes.

(2) There are differences between men and women in their willingness to report illness and behave as ill; in addition, it is socially more acceptable for women to be ill than it is for men.

(3) The sick role is more compatible with women's other roles, and hence easier for women to adopt than it is for men.

The first of these explanatory models concentrates on illness and assumes that illness and illness behaviour are the same thing. This is the one which most closely adheres to the medical model. In contrast the other two acknowledge that they are addressing illness behaviour only. It is beyond the scope of this book to examine the arguments in depth, but it is useful to consider two interesting studies which have implications for mental health and which lend support to the second and third models. Doyal (1979) has argued that it is unspoken, yet orthodox medical "knowledge" that men are normal and healthy and women are "abnormal" and hence unhealthy. She quotes an American study which asked doctors to describe a healthy adult (sex unspecified), a healthy man and a healthy woman. The medical views were that there was little difference between the first two, but that the healthy woman differed markedly towards more submissiveness, emotionality and less ambition. It also seemed that when asked to describe a healthy adult the doctors tended to think of a stereotyped male adult. Illness would seem to be less of a deviation from the norm for women and hence perhaps less stigmatising than it is for men.

In looking specifically at the sex differences in mental illness

Chesler (1974) has described various factors that she believes contribute to the higher rates for women, including oppression of women, their "expendability" in middle age, and women's conditioned role of help-seeking and distress-reporting leading to their greater willingness to adopt the sick role. She too agrees that "the ethic of mental health in our society is a masculine one".

Marriage

Although being married appears to give some protection to both sexes so that the rates of mental illness among married people are lower than they are for the divorced, widowed or single, the degree of the protection is very different for men and women (Table 2.1). The highest rate of mental illness for all groups is for single men, with the group least at risk being married men (Cochrane, 1983). The difference in the rates for married and single women is not nearly so striking, with only a slightly lower rate for the former. Indeed it is only among the married that the rates of reported mental ill-health become higher for women than for men. Among single people men have a higher rate of mental illness than do women.

Table 2.1   RATES OF ADMISSION TO MENTAL HOSPITAL PER 100 000 POPULATION BY SEX AND MARITAL STATUS, ENGLAND AND WALES, 1973

Marital status	Males	Females	Ratio M:F
Single	663	623	1:0.93
Married	257	433	1:1.68
Widowed	752	720	1:0.96
Divorced	1959	1596	1:0.81

Source: Cochrane, 1983.

Cochrane suggests a possible explanation for these marital differences by pointing out that women's roles may change more dramatically with marriage, and perhaps motherhood, than men's do, with all the consequent stress and possible frustration. Such an explanation is supported by health surveys which show that housewives are more likely than women who are employed outside the home to complain of psychiatric symptoms and to have tranquillisers and sleeping tablets prescribed (Waldron, 1980).

Other writers (for example, Oakley, 1974) have commented on the stress related to housework and found that housewives feel socially isolated and see themselves as having low prestige. The idea that housewives face greater stress would appear to support the first model mentioned above in that it suggests that housewives do indeed suffer from more mental ill-health rather than simply being more able to report it or to adopt the sick role. No single model based on gender and marital status appears then to be able to explain on its own the differences in detected mental ill-health rates. What is most likely is that all of the various influences act together to cause higher rates of mental ill-health and mental ill-health reporting in women.

When we consider the combined effect of gender and marital status, it is clear that it is of great significance for the work of CPNs. In our study in Bloomsbury health district, as might be expected from what was said above, we found that a disproportionate number of single, divorced and widowed people were referred to the CPN service (Brooker and Simmons, 1985). This has implications for the types of intervention that may be used by CPNs, and the kinds of skills that are needed for these perhaps isolated individuals. We shall return to this in a later chapter.

Social class and residential area

A number of studies have demonstrated a link between lower socioeconomic status and a higher risk of psychological problems, particularly in the field of schizophrenia. Several studies (for example, Faris and Dunham, 1939) have discovered that psychiatric disorder is far higher in the sometimes decaying inner-city areas than in the wealthier suburbs. Certainly, in our experience, in an inner-city health district, data collected on all those referred to the CPN service during 1984 show that a larger proportion than would be expected from national and local averages are living in rented accommodation or hostels, and rely on state support for their income. Both of these are indicators of lower socioeconomic status. Two main types of explanations for the differences in the rates of schizophrenia have been put forward: social causation and social selection.

Social causation theory argues that different factors in people's social situations – for example, poor housing, less pleasant working conditions and a lack of control over events in one's life – contribute to greater stress for certain sections of our society and hence lead to greater mental ill-health. Social selection theory is sometimes known as the "drift hypothesis" and suggests that those with schizophrenia in particular lose their social and occupational standing as a result of their illness (Goldberg and Morrison, 1963). It is sometimes suggested that this drift may happen over several generations. Certainly it seems likely that as a result of interpersonal and intellectual difficulties some of those with diagnoses of chronic schizophrenia may not be able to continue working as before. In addition, it is thought that a proportion of those who adopt an itinerant lifestyle and drift between inner city hostels may also be schizophrenics who have refused or have not had access to treatment.

It seems most likely that both these explanations are partially true, in that social drift does occur for individuals and perhaps families, but that life for those with less interesting and rewarding occupations, lower incomes and substandard housing is also inherently more stressful than it is for those who are better off.

There has also been interest among researchers in an examination of a possible link between mental ill-health and specific types of housing (see, for example, Taylor and Chave, 1964; Hare and Shaw, 1965; Fanning, 1967). New housing estates with the associated upheaval of families from older, possibly rundown, areas; new towns which may cause isolation, loneliness and "transitional neurosis" in those who move there; and high-rise blocks of flats, which have led to particularly high levels of dissatisfaction in families with young children, have all been implicated as contributing to stress and psychological problems. However, despite widespread agreement that such housing may contribute to mental health problems, the results of some of the research studies are somewhat conflicting and ambiguous. Fortunately many housing authorities have now changed their policies regarding the housing of families so that those with young children are now less likely to live high in a tower block.

Unemployment

Although unemployment is not, in theory at least, confined to one socioeconomic group, it tends to hit hardest people in semiskilled and unskilled occupations. In our society and as a result of our socialisation, work provides us with several benefits in addition to a regular income. These can be summarised as:

- A source of identity.
- A source of relationships outside the nuclear family (and, in addition, temporary acceptable distancing from the family).
- A source of obligatory activity (thus preventing prolonged inactivity).
- An opportunity to develop skills and creativity.
- Structuring of time.
- A sense of purpose which enhances self-esteem.
  (adapted from Fagin and Little, 1984).

Different types of work may give a person all or some of these, while the work of some people may also give them high status, job satisfaction, and an opportunity for self-actualisation. Clearly, many of these work-related benefits are intimately linked to a person's mental health. It is, therefore, not surprising that various writers have linked unemployment with increased levels of psychological problems, higher rates of self-injury and in some cases suicide. (Retirement, however, does not appear to have the same impact since it is more socially acceptable.) One study which looked at depression in young people found that those who were unemployed were more depressed than those in apprenticeships, and that young people on Youth Opportunities Schemes (YOPS) were only slightly less depressed than their unemployed peers (Branthwaite and Garcia, 1985). The researchers suggest that this was connected, not with the nature of the job, but with the uncertainty of the future for the YOPS participants.

Some researchers (for example, Cochrane, 1983) argue that being unemployed is one of the main determinants of poor mental health, especially for men. Women may be less affected by unemployment because of the availability of alternative acceptable roles such as motherhood (although women have higher rates of mental ill-health overall).

Fagin and Little (1984) carried out in-depth interviews with 22 families in which the male breadwinner had become unemployed in the previous 6–12 months. They looked at unemployment as a life-event or psychosocial transition that could affect all the members of the family. Four phases that an unemployed person may experience are described, these being similar to the stages of bereavement:

- Disbelief and shock.
- Denial and sometimes optimism – this may contribute to a "holiday" attitude.
- Anxiety and distress, as redundancy money runs out and no further employment is found.
- Resignation and adjustment – adopting a non-occupational identity; in this stage the whole family may change its standards and expectations.

In fact the researchers found that the first and second stages were very rare in their interviewees, and that the third stage of anxiety and depression was the most frequently experienced. Health problems were very common in the families, with complaints of depression, suicidal thoughts, psychosomatic disorders, increased cigarette smoking and changes in the health of the children. Fagin and Little also suggest that there could be an increased risk of child abuse. They postulate that the increased levels of illness may result from the sick role being more acceptable to the men and their families than the role of long-term unemployed. This is not, they argue, a conscious choice, but one that arises from the values of our society. They conclude by recommending economic and educational changes, but they also stress the need for counselling and for the families to have someone who will listen to them. They found that their interviews provided an opportunity for family members to talk to each other in a way that, in some cases, they had not done for months.

Stress and life-events

Many studies have shown that high levels of stress and negative life-events can lead to an increased risk of mental illness. (Life-events are discussed more fully in Chapter 4.) It is thought that stress is the link between such life-events, environmental factors and so on and physical and mental ill-health. The negative impact of such stressors appears to be particularly high where they are experienced in isolation – for instance in the case of marital breakdown or redundancy. Where extremely traumatic events have an impact on a whole community – such as in wartime – the incidence of mental hospital admission and suicide actually falls. Perhaps even more surprising, the symptoms may be more likely to persist if the person is removed from the scene of danger rather than kept with the environment he knows. One plausible explanation is that the experiences bring people closer together, and the negative impact is counteracted by increased community cohesiveness (Coser, 1956). Studies that have looked at individuals' reactions to the stress of living through the "troubles" in Northern Ireland suggest that there is an acute emotional reaction which is usually quickly resolved. However, in areas peripheral to the scenes of greatest rioting there is indeed an increase in mental ill-health, indicating that it may be the associated anxiety, not the actual violent experience, that is the main stressor (Fraser, 1974; Lyons, 1972).

The link between life-events and depression in women has been examined by comparing a sample of in-patients and a group of women randomly selected from the local community (Brown and Harris, 1978). The study found that 30% of the comparison group had some psychological problems according to their criteria, and that the most common problem was depression, often associated with the loss of a "significant other" by death or separation, or with the loss of home or employment. By examining the fabric of the women's lives, Brown and Harris were able to identify four factors that they concluded increased the likelihood of a woman developing depression in response to such life stresses:

● No paid employment.
● An absence of an intimate, confiding relationship with the woman's husband or boyfriend.
● Three or more children under 14 living at home.
● An early loss of her own mother.

They also found that just as her own employment may afford a woman some protection, unemployment in her husband appears to increase the likelihood of a woman having mental health problems.

Cultural and ethnic differences

The concept of mental illness (as opposed to witchcraft, possession by evil spirits, special religious powers etc.) has not been consistent throughout earlier centuries, although Clare (1976) points out that there have been long periods (going back to Hippocrates) when psychiatric disturbance was considered natural rather than supernatural. Similarly, it is not always present in the same form in other cultures. Behaviour which in our society would be diagnosed as schizophrenic does appear in individuals in other societies but may be interpreted quite differently (Cochrane, 1983). Where it is thought of as temporary, the sufferers appear to recover more quickly and perhaps completely. In contrast, in our society, where schizophrenia is often thought of as potentially long-term, total recovery is rarer. Similarly, depression and other neuroses are not considered as entities in some cultures. The same symptoms may be reported but they are not put together into a syndrome.

For nurses working in a multi-ethnic western society such as our own, perhaps the most important issue is to be aware, not necessarily of the details of cultural differences of all the ethnic groups encountered (since this would probably be impossible), but of the existence of these differences.

There are, of course, different degrees of integration into the native community among the different immigrant groups, and different rates of use of the psychiatric services. For example, the Irish are over-represented in terms of psychiatric admission, with Irish men often being admitted with alcohol-related problems. West Indians have a slightly higher rate of psychiatric hospital admission, a significantly higher frequency of diagnoses of schizophrenia (especially amongst men) and, in London at least, a much greater likelihood of compulsory admission under Section 136 of the 1983 Mental Health Act than the indigenous population (GLC, 1984). It is possible that schizophrenia may be overdiagnosed because of a lack of understanding of different kinds of cultural expression and poor communication with the person and his family. West Indians tend to have more "disturbed" illnesses, and hence are perhaps more likely to be admitted than those who become withdrawn when ill (Littlewood and Lipsedge, 1982). In some instances, however, the higher rates of admission could reflect the difficulty some groups have in gaining access to, or making use of, primary mental health care at an earlier stage. Just as schizophrenia may be overdiagnosed, depression may be missed in people from different cultures where distress may be expressed through physical symptoms more often than it is in the majority group.

However, as the GLC report points out, it would be wrong to assume that those from an ethnic minority will inevitably have more problems than the majority population since Indians, Chinese and Italians generally have lower admission rates. One possibility is that this could reflect the existence of more cohesive networks in these cultures, rather than a major difference in levels of psychiatric problems.

Once in the in-patient or out-patient treatment services, the black person may experience another difference in the types of therapy offered, according to the GLC report. Black and ethnic minority people are more likely to receive physical treatment, including electroconvulsive therapy and drugs, where white people may be offered psychotherapy. (This may, however, be more of a class than a racial difference since black people are, in British society, more likely to be working class, and it has been reported that working-class people in general are less likely to receive psychotherapy than are middle-class people.)

Just as we talked earlier about the higher rates of stress in the lower socioeconomic groups, we can also expect that the level of stress will be higher among groups who have left their own society to join one which is at times hostile, where their own language is seldom heard outside their home, and where their prospects of employment may be poor. New immigrants to this country tend to find housing in the sometimes rundown parts of the cities where there is a high turnover in the residential population. In the 1950s the London boroughs with the greatest in-migration and out-migration had the highest suicide rates (Sainsbury, 1955). Although it would be misleading to assume that those people who have recently moved to an area are also the ones who kill themselves, this study does suggest that a high level of stress exists in such environments.

In examining the figures from the 1971 National Census Littlewood and Lipsedge (1982, p. 129) write that:

> There is abundant evidence that material and environmental deprivation is experienced by ethnic minority groups. The West Indian community in particular experiences overcrowding and shared dwellings, lack of amenities, high unemployment and low family incomes.

They also conclude that some of the emotional difficulties that are experienced by immigrants may be related to discrimination and racism within the psychiatric services as well as in society as a whole.

Until recently mental health services have made no special provision for those from different ethnic backgrounds, but there is a growing realisation that this is needed. It is also now recognised that it is not enough simply to attempt to increase access to already existing services, including CPN teams, where these services may be mainly geared towards the native white population. We may need to establish different types of services employing people as mental health workers who are themselves from the same ethnic groups as the local community or, if this is not possible in the short-term, increase the employment of interpreters.

The Changing Nature of Our Society
Family life

Enormous changes in the structure and organisation of western society have taken place since the Industrial Revolution. One of the most far-reaching of these has been in the pattern of family life. It is generally accepted by sociologists and anthropologists that the family as the main primary group is fairly universal to societies throughout the world, although the patterns of family organisation may vary widely, both within one community and between different societies. Generally family members live together, pool their resources and jointly produce and raise children.

In examining the work of sociologists in this field, Haralambos (1980) makes the point that many of the writers on the role and functions of the family have started from a particular ideological position which has been elaborated through their writing. Some hold a strong belief that the family should be fostered and encouraged. For example, Haralambos quotes the sociologist Murdock, who has described four functions of the family that he says serve the needs of individual family members and society as a whole: sexual, reproductive, economic, and educational (including socialisation). Talcott Parsons outlines only two functions, the primary socialisation of children and the stabilisation of adult personalities (see Haralambos, 1980). The latter is provided through the marital relationship which, through the giving of emotional support, counteracts the stresses of everyday life. Such a suggestion would appear to be partially supported by Brown and Harris's work, referred to earlier, which found that the existence of a close, confiding adult relationship, which may or may not be with a spouse, offered some protection against depression in women.

However, there have been strong criticisms of such a rosy view of family life from writers who see the family as potentially destructive rather than supportive of its members. Such criticisms have come from the women's liberation movement which has argued that women are exploited by the family structure; and from within psychiatry, for example Laing (1976b) and Cooper (1972) who say that interaction within the family pushes children into making impossible choices and prevents them from developing their own individuality.

Certainly it seems likely that neither view of family life adequately portrays the wide variety of family organisation and patterns of communication that we may find in a society containing many different socioeconomic and ethnic groups. Both descriptions could be said to be of the extremes while most families, as CPNs will be only too aware, will fall somewhere along a continuum with varying and changing advantages and disadvantages for their members.

The pattern of family life has been studied in great depth by Young and Wilmott (1962 and 1975). They have identified four stages through which communities may move, two of which are of particular importance to people like CPNs who work with families. They describe stage 2 family structure as coming about during the Industrial Revolution, but say that although it has largely died out now it may still be found in low-income, well-established working-class areas where there has been little geographical mobility. In these families the bond between the wife and her mother is stronger than that between wife and husband, and the female members of the family see each other frequently, exchange services (for example, shopping and child care) and socialise together. The husband is fairly peripheral to the family, and may spend a lot of time outside the home. Although it is unlikely that we would now find all the features of Young and Wilmott's description in a single family, CPNs will indeed come into contact with some families with some of these characteristics.

Young and Wilmott's stage 3 family organisation is now the most common. In this family the husband plays a more central role, and the household tasks are shared by husband and wife, although their roles will not generally be interchangeable. Family life is more home-based, especially among working-class families.

There is general agreement among most writers that the family has lost some of its original functions, such as the education of children and care of sick members, with the introduction of the educational system and the health and social services. The increasingly specialised functions of the family have led to a greater emotional intensity, interdependence and isolation from the wider society. When greater emotional support is available within a family, its members may derive a sense of wholeness and permanence, but when individual needs are not met there may be greater strain and less access to a wider network which could defuse the problems. It is not true, however, that the family has lost the functions of health care completely. In most cases of illness the primary care is indeed still provided by members of the family, and (as we shall see later) there is evidence that this caring role of the family in relation to sick or elderly members may be further encouraged or even expected by the state.

There is, we think, another major shortcoming of these analyses of the family in that they concentrate on one particular family model – the nuclear family of two parents and their children. Although this may be the most common form of family organisation, it is quite misleading to think that most people live in such a family system. In fact when we examine all those who live in private households we find just under half live in a household made up of a married couple and dependent children. Other types of private household include those living alone, couples without children and multi-family households. The number of people who live alone has risen from 4% in 1961 to 9% in 1982, the increase being mostly accounted for by the larger numbers of elderly people (women over 60 and men over 65) of whom 30% live alone (Central Statistical Office, 1984). At the same time there has been, during the twentieth century, a steady rise in the rate of marital breakdown, to the extent that for every three marriages in the 1970s there was one divorce. This rate is higher for marriages where one or both partners are teenagers at the time of marriage, or have been married before. The higher rates of divorce have lead to more single-parent households or, in the case of remarriage, more step-families, where the children are from previous relationships.

Old people

There have been other major changes in the pattern of our society over the past decades. One of the most striking of these is in the age distribution of the population. Generally, the population is getting older. There are two main reasons for this. First, the birth rate has fallen (although it is now beginning to rise again towards another "baby boom"). Second, life expectancy has increased, so that there are more people living into old age. The population of the United Kingdom has been relatively stable since 1971, but there have been changes in its composition, with a lower proportion being children and a higher proportion being elderly (the number of people of pensionable age rose by a million between 1971 and 1981). It is expected that the population will now rise only very slightly up to the end of the century. Within this population it is predicted that the number of people over 65 will not increase markedly beyond the 1981 level, but the proportion of these who are very elderly will increase. To illustrate this, currently the over-85 age-group make up approximately 7% of the elderly population; in 2001 they will make up 12% (Central Statistical Office, 1984).

It is these very elderly people who are likely to make most demands on the health and social services and, as a result of isolation, bereavement, psychological problems related to poorer physical health, and, in some instances, organic psychiatric conditions, to require greater community mental health care. The Health Advisory Service (1982) suggests that the great majority of old people with mental illness will remain at home under the care of their general practitioners, with the support of social and community health services.

When we consider organic conditions in particular, the Health Advisory Service estimates that 10% of those over 65, rising to 20% of those over 80, show some evidence of dementia. This report also notes that family support is less available than it has been in the past, although most old people are still living in their own homes. Abrams (1980) would agree with this. He found in his survey that half of all women over 75 lived alone (women constituted two-thirds of all those aged 75 and over), and that this group were twice as likely to suffer from feelings of loneliness, uselessness and frustration than those living with others. It is also salutary to remember that suicide rates among old people are higher, indeed twice as high for the over 65s as for the under 35s. Elderly men are especially at risk.

To summarise so far, we have presented in this chapter some of the main theoretical and demographic themes of the book. These include some sociological concepts relevant to mental health, such as labelling theory, the theory of role and status, and the relationship between certain social variables and mental illness. We have also discussed the changing pattern of our society. We shall now briefly look at some of the social policies that have affected mental health services.

Social and Mental Health Policy

We would now like to consider some of the policy background to the growth and development of community mental health services. The particular growth of CPN services will be dealt with more fully in the next chapter.

It is helpful to understand something of the economic constraints that affect planning at district and regional levels. The resources of the NHS have been until the past few years distributed rather unevenly over the country, so that some areas, particularly the teaching districts and the South-east, have been richer than others. Indeed, the expression "inverse care law" was coined to describe this situation where "the availability of good medical care tends to vary inversely with the need of the population served" (Tudor Hart, 1971). In 1976 the Resource Allocation Working Party (RAWP) drew up recommendations for the gradual reallocation of these resources to arrive at a service that would provide equal opportunity of access to health care for people at equal risk (DHSS, 1976). The working party started from the premise that demand for health care will always exceed resources and that the supply of health care fuels demand. They also acknowledged that disparities of provision could not be corrected at a single stroke, and recommended that funding should gradually be transferred from the "over-resourced" regions to the "under-resourced" ones by a process of fixing growth targets at different levels.

The criteria of need used to determine the allocations to individual regions and districts include population size and make-up (sex, age), morbidity, differential costs of care, education needs, and capital investment. In terms of psychiatric care, the working party looked only at in-patient services and recommended that the particular population's composition by age, sex and marital status, be used as the main criteria, since as we have seen these variables have been recognised as significant in predicting the use of psychiatric services. The working party also considered other variables, including class, poverty and degree of isolation, but recommended that further research was needed to determine the effect of these.

Parallel to these changes in NHS resource allocations, there were also changes taking place in policies affecting the provision of mental health services. The growth and development of community psychiatric nursing services are very much part of an overall shift, during the past decades, in the type of care being provided for people with mental health problems. It is important that we recognise the part played by official policy in reflecting, responding to and at times formalising this changing philosophy of care.

The 1959 Mental Health Act aimed at the minimisation of institutional care and allowed for community-based care and treatment to be developed. Following this the Ministry of Health (1962) set out plans for the rundown and possible closure of large mental hospitals, with care to be provided by units in district general hospitals (DGHs) and in the community. Despite such policies, however, the development of community-based services was somewhat patchy. By the mid-1970s there was a growing consensus that there should be more attempts to reintegrate into the community people who have had psychiatric admissions, rather than keeping them in institutions (Gostin, 1975). It was acknowledged that the longer someone remained in hospital, the more likely it was that he would become institutionalised and that there would almost certainly be a deterioration in his mental state and level of functioning. Gostin's report, which argued for a revision of the Mental Health Act, concluded that: "no person should be admitted to a treatment facility unless a prior determination is made that the facility is the least restrictive setting necessary for that person".

At almost the same time, the Department of Health and Social Security brought out a major report on the future provision of psychiatric care, *Better Services for the Mentally Ill* (DHSS, 1975). This report acknowledged that there had been some moves towards community care in the 1950s and 1960s, and welcomed the setting up of some psychiatric units in district general hospitals.

The main proposals of the report concerned the need to establish flexible and local services in which the care and treatment of those with long-term mental illness would be integrated with treatment for those with short-term problems. However, the document recognised that the policy of increasing the accessibility and flexibility of mental health services, combined with the trend within society to push back the boundaries of what is mental ill-health, could have major implications. In considering this the report says "We must recognise that the potential demand for psychiatric help is virtually unlimited" (DHSS, 1975, p. 1), and argues that the provision for long-term patients must not be a second-tier, under-resourced service.

The DHSS outlined the type of service needed by pointing out that a great deal of psychiatric care is provided by primary health care teams and that support from a specialist team, working with a community orientation, should provide back-up. The specialist team would include CPNs and other professionals and would form a part of the comprehensive service which would encompass: a DGH psychiatric unit; day hospital; facilities for elderly people; social services input (including day and residential care, social clubs); care of long-term mentally ill people; and facilities for the homeless and rootless population. At the time of the document it was not government policy to close or run down large mental hospitals, but to first replace them with a better, local range of services. The report made the point that even when these services were developed it would not be appropriate to close hospitals if they were still required for residents who had been admitted many years earlier and could not be resettled in the community.

Better Services for the Mentally Ill also stressed the need for the joint planning of psychiatric services between health authorities and local authority social services departments. The mechanism for this, the Joint Consultative Committees, made up of representatives from both organisations, had already been set up by the NHS Reorganisation Act,

In 1983 another step was taken in the direction of a different pattern of mental health care in this country with the revised Mental Health Act. The Act adopts the principle of the "least restrictive alternative" to hospital admission, and thus stresses the need for community facilities (Gostin, 1983). Yet another step was taken with many regional health authorities drawing up plans for the actual closure of one or more large psychiatric hospitals and the parallel development of alternative services.

Chapter 3 examines the specific development of community psychiatric nursing services. We shall also return to many of this chapter's themes, and the relevance of this wider perspective to the delivery of good community psychiatric nursing care, in later sections of the book.

References

Abrams, M. (1980). *Beyond Three-score and Ten*, 2nd report. Age Concern Publications, Mitcham.

Banton, M. (1965). *Roles*. Tavistock, London.

Becker, H. S. (1963). *Outsiders: Studies in the Sociology of Deviance*. Free Press, Glencoe.

Branthwaite, A. and Garcia, S. (1985). Depression in the young unemployed and those on Youth Opportunities Schemes. *British Journal of Medical Psychology*, **58**: 67–74.

Brooker, C. and Simmons, S. (1985). A study to compare two models of community psychiatric nursing care delivery. *Journal of Advanced Nursing*, **10**: 217–23.

Brown, G. W. and Harris, T. O. (1978). *The Social Origins of Depression*. Tavistock, London.

Central Statistical Office (1984). *Social Trends* 14. HMSO, London.

Chesler, P. (1974). *Women and Madness*. Allen Lane, London.

Clare, A. (1976). *Psychiatry in Dissent*. Tavistock, London.

Cochrane, R. (1983). *The Social Creation of Mental Illness*. Longman, London.

Cooper, D. (1972). *The Death of the Family*. Penguin, Harmondsworth.

Cooper, J. E., Kendell, R. E., Gurland, B. J., Sharpe, L., Copeland, J. R. M., and Simon, R. J. (1972). *Psychiatric Diagnosis in New York and London*. Oxford University Press, London.

Coser, L. A. (1956). *The Functions of Conflict*. The Free Press, Glencoe.

DHSS (1975). *Better Services for the Mentally Ill*. Cmnd 6233, HMSO, London.

DHSS (1976). *Sharing Resources for Health in England: Report of the Resource Allocation Working Party*. HMSO, London.

Dingwall, R. (1976). *Aspects of Illness*. Martin Robertson, London.

Doyal, L. (1979). *The Political Economy of Health*. Pluto Press, London.

Fagin, L. and Little, M. (1984). *The Forsaken Families*. Penguin, Harmondsworth.

Fanning, D. M. (1967). Families in flats. *British Medical Journal*, **4**: 382–6.

Faris, R. E. L. and Dunham, H. W. (1939). *Mental Disorders in Urban Areas*. Chicago University Press, Chicago.

Fraser, M. (1974). *Children in Conflict*. Penguin, Harmondsworth.

GLC (1984). *Mental Health Services in London*. GLC, London.

Goffman, E. (1961). *Asylums*. Penguin, Harmondsworth.

Goldberg, E. M. and Morrison, S. C. (1963). Schizophrenia and social class. *British Journal of Psychiatry*, **109**: 785–802.

Gostin, L. (1975). *A Human Condition*. MIND, London.

Gostin, L. (1983). *A Practical Guide to Mental Health Law*. MIND, London.

Hare, E. H. and Shaw, G. K. (1965). *Mental Health on a New Housing Estate*. Oxford University Press, Oxford.

Haralambos, M. (1980). *Sociology: Themes and Perspectives*. University Tutorial Press, Slough.

Health Advisory Service (1982). *The Rising Tide – Developing Services for Mental Illness in Old Age*. Health Advisory Service, Surrey.

Horne, M. (1985). A word in your head. *Nursing Mirror*, **160**(23): 34–5.

Ineichen, B. (1979). *Mental Illness*. Longman, London.

Laing, R. D. (1976a). *The Facts of Life*. Allen Lane, London.

Laing, R. D. (1976b). *The Politics of the Family*. Penguin, Harmondsworth.

Littlewood, R. and Lipsedge, M. (1982). *Aliens and Alienists: Ethnic Minorities and Psychiatry*. Penguin, Harmondsworth.

Lyons, H. A. (1972). Depressive illness and aggression in Belfast. *British Medical Journal*, 1: 324–4.

Mangen, S. P. (1982). *Sociology and Mental Health*. Churchill Livingstone, Edinburgh.

MIND (1980). *Mental Health Statistics*. MIND, London.

Ministry of Health (1962). *A Hospital Plan for England and Wales*. Cmnd 1604, HMSO, London.

Nathanson, C. (1978). Sex roles as variables in the interpretation of morbidity data: a methodological critique. *International Journal of Epidemiology*, 7(3): 253–62.

Oakley, A. (1974). *The Sociology of Housework*. Martin Robertson, London.

Robinson, D. (1971). *The Process of Becoming Ill*. Routledge and Kegan Paul, London.

Rosenhan, D. L. (1979). On being sane in insane places, in Whitten, P. (ed.) *Readings in Sociology: Contemporary Perspectives*. Harper and Row, New York.

Sainsbury, P. (1955). *Suicide in London*. Chapman and Hall, London.

Scheff, T. (1966). *Being Mentally Ill*. Weidenfeld and Nicolson, London.

Taylor, L. and Chave, S. (1964). *Mental Health and Environment*. Longman, London.

Tudor Hart, J. (1971). The inverse care law. *Lancet*, 1: 405–12.

Waldron, I. (1980). Employment and women's health: an analysis of causal relationships. *International Journal of Health Services*, 10(3): 435–54.

Young, M. and Willmott, P. (1962). *Family and Kinship in East London*. Penguin, Harmondsworth.

Young, M. and Willmott, P. (1975). *The Symmetrical Family*. Penguin, Harmondsworth.

3

The Organisation of CPN Services

Introduction

Since the first CPN service was established in 1954, community psychiatric nursing has become one of the largest growth areas in the mental health service. That CPN services have developed so rapidly is a success story requiring some explanation. Fortunately, much has been written about the CPN's rise over the past 30 years, and this volume of writing reflects the great enthusiasm which has greeted this branch of psychiatric nursing.

Certain unique conditions prevailed in the 1950s that gave rise to the first CPN service. At that time psychiatric nurses had a purely custodial role and worked exclusively on hospital wards. Henderson (1945, p. 68) described the role of the psychiatric nurse as: "cleanliness, order, punctuality, discipline, attention to detail, observation, and what to report to the doctor, collectively they are the basis of good mental nursing." Psychiatric nursing was little different from general nursing, indeed there were theatre nurses in psychiatric hospitals whose entire role was to assist at leucotomy operations. Psychiatric patients were never sent to any other hospital, all their health needs being met within the institution.

However, a major revolution was on the horizon. In 1952, Delay and Deniker described for the first time the pharmacological action of a drug to be marketed under the trade name "Largactil". Largactil and the other major tranquillisers proved to be exceptionally valuable antipsychotic agents, alleviating delusions, hallucinations and disturbed behaviour particularly in people diagnosed as schizophrenic. The phenothiazines reduced bizarre schizophrenic symptoms to the point where sufferers became much more amenable to "social" and "interpersonal" intervention. The nurse–patient relationship became a reality, and for the first time nurses were able to work with patients to plan their discharge home.

The drug revolution also meant that the length of a patient's stay in hospital became shorter and that it was now feasible to discharge people who had been in hospital for many years. Consequently, the numbers of people occupying beds in psychiatric hospitals declined dramatically from 154 000 in 1954 to 105 000 in 1976 (Royal Commission on NHS, 1979).

The 1950s also saw a fundamental change in attitudes to the mentally ill, as enshrined by statute in the 1959 Mental Health Act. This Act repealed the 1930 Mental Treatment Act which had reinforced the segregation of people with mental illness from the public. The spirit of the 1959 Act was very different as it aimed to strengthen community links; for example, involuntary admission to hospital required the involvement of GPs and social workers.

A recent government inquiry into community care for the mentally ill has succinctly summarised these developments:

> In the 1950s the pace of reform gathered, as a result of the introduction of drugs (such as reserpine and chlorpromazine), social treatments, and the Royal Commission on mental illness and mental deficiency of 1954–7, culminating in the 1959 Mental Health Act. The phrase "community care" occurred in policy statements with increasing frequency. (House of Commons Social Services Select Committee, 1985, para 14.)

"Care in the community" for people with mental illness became a clarion call for those who advocated a more socially oriented model of mental health care.

Such was the dramatic and sudden change in emphasis in mental health provision that in 1961 Tooth and Brook, two government statisticians, stated that: "Between 1955 and 1959, the long stay population resident on the 31st December, 1954, was running down at such a rate, which if continued, would eliminate it in about sixteen years." With the benefit of hindsight we now know that this forecast was overly optimistic but at the time their paper was hugely influential. Many argue that Tooth and Brook's statistical analysis provided the momentum for the 1962 Government White Paper *The Hospital Plan*. This document (see Chapter 2) was the forerunner of much subsequent government policy directed at closing large Victorian institutions and replacing them with community care initiatives.

This then is the wider mental health world into which the CPN service was born and in which CPN services grew rapidly. In the following two sections we trace the development of the CPN "child" into young adulthood from 1945 to 1979; during this phase CPN services grew slowly, struggled, experimented and gradually acquired a more sophisticated role. We shall then examine how the organisation of the CPN team changed during the years 1980–85. Much of our information comes from the Community Psychiatric Nursing Association (CPNA). This group carried out two major surveys in 1980 and 1985 which examined nationally the major aspects of CPN services. These surveys provide key information on issues such as the volume of the CPN workforce, the grades on which they are employed, the bases they use, and from whom they gain their referrals.

Community Psychiatric Nursing: The Early Years 1954–79

1954–70

The first CPN service established in this country was at Warlingham Park Hospital, Surrey, in 1954. Two nurses were seconded from their usual ward duties to work in the catchment area day hospital in Croydon. They worked with patients discharged from the parent hospital, and their role was initially very basic. They visited patients at home, ensured that they were taking medication, made a nursing assessment of the patient's mental state, and discussed the patient's overall treatment programme with relatives. These early CPNs also attended out-patient clinics and ran evening social club groups and recreational activities. All their initiatives were supervised by the community psychiatrist at a formal weekly meeting (May and Moore, 1963).

Lena Peat, one of these first CPNs, says that the impetus for the new service came from a hospital consultant psychiatrist who felt that psychiatric nurses ought to broaden their horizons beyond the hospital gates (Peat and Watt, 1984). She also describes how the original CPNs rotated every six months from their duties in the community back to more conventional work as ward sisters. However, the drawbacks of that arrangement were soon realised, and the "out-patient" nurses were working full-time in the community within a year. Peat also comments that the development of the role was firmly in line with Warlingham Park Hospital's "open-door" policy.

The only other service established in the 1950s was at Moorhaven Hospital, Devon, in 1957 (Hunter, 1974). Like its counterpart in Surrey it was originally called a "nursing after-care" service and not a CPN service. Unlike Surrey, however, the Moorhaven CPN service gave the CPN a role similar in status to that of the social worker: the Moorhaven CPN was expected to build a relationship with the patient and was clearly seen to be a therapeutic agent in his or her own right. It is useful to note that Hunter's description of the CPN's role is very similar to the model of psychiatric nursing outlined by Peplau in 1952.

In both these early services, psychiatric nurses began working in the community on a part-time basis; at Moorhaven the nurses worked for part of the week in the hospital, and it was recognised that the patients would continue to be dependent on the hospital. This part-time pattern of provision predominated at least until the mid-1960s; in 1966 an RCN survey found that 42 hospitals employed CPNs but that, out of a total workforce of 225 nurses, only 26 were working full-time in a community setting (RCN, 1966).

1970–79

In 1970 the Local Authorities Act was implemented and had a huge impact on the expansion of CPN services. It incorporated the main recommendations of the Seebohm Report (1968) by absorbing local authority mental health departments and mental welfare officers into generic social service departments. Thus, mental health became the concern of all social workers and not just the specially trained psychiatric social workers. As Paykel and Griffiths (1983, p. 10) have pointed out: "Specialised workers were temporarily replaced by relatively inexperienced generalist social workers with different skills and priorities leaving a vacuum in follow-up care."

There was clearly a need for a new group of community-oriented mental health professionals to fill the gap created by the local government reorganisation. This need was felt across the professional groups. For example the Royal Medico-Psychological Association (now the Royal College of Psychiatrists) stated in 1969: "It is likely that a new body of mental health social workers would have to be evolved to fill the gap left by the destruction of the present growing services, perhaps with an enhanced medical or nursing background." A psychiatric nurse manager in Oxford described the chaos that ensued at a psychiatric hospital after the creation of new social service departments (Leopoldt and Hurn, 1973). He argued that the problems could only be overcome if nurses could provide the social and rehabilitative care previously provided by the psychiatric social worker. We shall now show how community psychiatric nursing grew in the decade 1970–80 to meet the need for a new community-based mental health worker.

A large number of new CPN services were established during this 10-year period, the greatest number being set up in 1974 (see Fig. 3.1) (McKendrick, 1980). The number of full-time equivalent CPN posts rose from 663 in 1976 to 1667 in 1980.

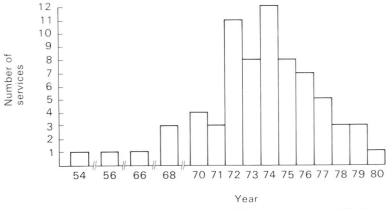

Fig. 3.1   Histogram of number of services established per year (*n* = 71). Source: McKendrick (1980).

As new CPN services took shape, and staffing levels within teams grew, so the individual roles of CPNs begun to diverge. Indeed, the increase in the CPN workforce engendered a new confidence to experiment with the traditional CPN role.

Most importantly, CPN team organisation began to evolve along two separate lines.

As far back as 1967, the World Health Organization had predicted that CPN services could develop in two different ways.

First, the service could be based in a psychiatric hospital, work within hospital treatment teams, accepting referrals exclusively from psychiatrists – in other words, operating a "closed" referral system. In the second model, CPNs could be attached to general practices or health clinics, in much the same way as are health visitors and district nurses; in this scenario, the CPNs would operate an "open" referral pattern, accepting referrals from any professional source, and indeed self-referrals from clients themselves.

By 1978 it was clear that there was a definite movement towards the open referral pattern (Parnell, 1978). In a paper in 1973, Leopoldt and Hurn described the first attachment of CPNs to general practice in the Oxford region and raised two major issues. First, the change in base for the CPN led to a change in role; the CPN became an independent practitioner, working in a relatively unsupported environment, responsible for the assessment and investigation of suspected mental health problems, aiming to establish and maintain a supportive role not just with the identified client but their family and friends as well and, in some cases, becoming responsible for establishing a programme of treatment or rehabilitation.

Second, Leopoldt and Hurn's article pointed out the inherent advantages of such a CPN organisational system as identified by the group practice team. The GPs referred readily to the CPN before crises occurred; in other words, crises were prevented from developing. This often led to the deferment of admission to psychiatric hospital. When admission did occur, however, communication about discharge was considerably facilitated as the CPN had a working knowledge of the hospital. Finally, the other practice nurses became much more confident about their own dealings with mental health problems, because they knew they could call upon the CPN's special knowledge.

Corser and Ryce (1977) describe a similar developing role for the CPN in a group practice in Scotland. The most significant finding here was the 97% attendance rate once clients had been referred to the sessional psychiatrist or CPN. This suggests that clients find this model of care relatively convenient and free from stigma.

Finally, more evidence of the growing popularity of the open referral system comes from a survey of CPN services undertaken in the North West Regional Health Authority in the 1970s (Shore, 1977). This study demonstrated that of the 17 CPN services in the Region, seven accepted referrals from consultant psychiatrists only or, to put it another way, seven services operated closed referral systems.

Of course the three studies referred to here are selective, and many more articles appeared in the 1970s which looked at experimental CPN attachments. (See Griffith and Mangen's 1980 literature review, especially pp. 201–2.) We feel it important to underline that CPN services in the 1970s were growing rapidly, growth led to experimentation in attachment, and a new work setting accompanied a change in the nature of a CPN's role.

The 1970s were a watershed for CPNs for another reason as well. They began to specialise for the first time, usually with a specific client group but sometimes with specialist functions, such as crisis intervention, within a multidisciplinary team (Strobie and Hopkins, 1972). In many ways CNP specialisation mirrored that of their consultant psychiatrist colleagues, and it is clear that often the case for CPN specialism was put most forcibly by psychiatrists. One good example of this is behaviour therapy. In 1972 the Department of Health and Social Security funded a three-year experimental research programme to examine the effectiveness of psychiatric nurses as the main therapists for a group of patients with selected "neurotic" conditions. This research led to approval by the Joint Board of Clinical Nursing Studies for an 18-month course in adult behavioural psychotherapy, under the direction of a psychiatrist, Professor I. Marks. The course is now designated "ENB cc no. 650" and over 75 nurses have graduated from it (Brooker and Brown, 1986).

When CPNs did specialise with a client group, it tended and still tends to be elderly mentally ill people. In Chapter 2, we showed the changes in the demography of the population. One of the most major of these has been in the increase of elderly people, and thus the number of elderly people with mental health problems. This fact combined with the generally poor local authority provision for elderly people and the lack of new appointments for consultant psychogeriatricians make this growing CPN specialisation highly appropriate. Aire and Isaacs (1978) give a good account of CPN involvement in a multidisciplinary team for elderly people in Essex. The CPNs were based in a health centre and operated an "open" referral system. Their main function was to give psychological support to family carers (and where necessary provide respite opportunities); however, practical nursing care was provided as well.

Other groups also began to receive specialist attention from CPNs during this period: children and adolescents, people with drug and alcohol problems, and former long-stay psychiatric patients who were being gradually relocated to community housing schemes.

In conclusion, we can note the following points: first, CPNs grew dramatically as a total workforce from four in 1954, to 226 in 1966, to some 1667 in 1980. This expansion, particularly in the 1970s, led to an increase in confidence in CPNs' views of their own abilities as therapeutic agents. The reorganisation of social service departments in 1970 provided an opportunity for psychiatric nurses to demonstrate their capabilities on a far wider scale. This opportunity was firmly grasped – CPNs changed the way their services were organised and ultimately their nursing role. CPN team organisation nationwide developed in an unstandardised way. There was a move away from the hospital to attachments in the community, and CPN specialism began to emerge.

The Organisation of CPN Services 1980–85

Two national CPNA-sponsored surveys of community psychiatric nursing were undertaken in 1980 and 1985. Prior to the first study in 1980, the CPNA explained why it was necessary: "There is a need to understand how services organise their delivery of care. The scanty information available on types of services, peripheral bases, attachment schemes and referral systems requires updating in order to provide a national picture."

Information was collected in three main areas – service organisation, total workforce figures and education. The 1980 survey's major findings were:

- Only six districts were without a CPN service in 1980.
- 25% of services worked in districts other than their own.
- Care of elderly people was the largest specialty – but was provided by only 18% of services.
- Over half of all CPN services were based in psychiatric hospitals.
- Regional variation in CPN staffing figures and population ratios demonstrated the absence of national norms and reflected local priority.

- Most services had a nursing officer managing the team.
- Not more than 20% of practising CPNs held the JBCNS certificate no. 800/810 in community psychiatric nursing.
- 25% of CPN teams accepted referrals from consultant psychiatrists only.

As this appears to be a relatively clear description of CPN organisation in 1980, why was the survey repeated in 1985? The answer is that rapid changes in the mental health service, particularly the run-down and projected closures of the big psychiatric hospitals, created a need for accurate and up-to-date information about CPN services.

In March 1985, the great need for a follow-up survey was stressed by the *Nursing Times* in an editorial about the Short Report into community care (HMSO, 1985):

> Above all, however, this report exposes a lack of leadership and direction from the DHSS and considerable apprehension and uncertainty at local levels as to the future pattern of provision. As the Committee acknowledged "the frontiers are still relatively unexplored". All the more reason for advice and support from the centre, for already the hospital population has fallen 21 000 to 69 000 in the past decade. The Government meanwhile doesn't know even how many CPNs there are, let alone how many there ought to be.

The 1985 CPNA survey remedied this situation: Furthermore, it was designed to allow comparisons with the 1980 situation. The following is an examination of the changes in CPN organisation during the period 1980–85, using these two surveys as our information source.

The CPN Workforce 1980–85

The total workforce

Table 3.1 shows the total CPN workforce figures by grade of nurse and compares the situation nationally in both 1980 and 1985. The most important finding is the rapid growth in the number of CPNs. In 1980 there were 1667 CPNs; by 1985 this figure had risen by 65% to a total of 2758.

This growth, however, is not consistent across all grades of staff. There has, for example, been a decrease in the use of the Nursing Officer grade (or its equivalent) – with 82 fewer posts at

Table 3.1 TOTAL WORKFORCE FIGURES BY GRADE AND YEAR

Grade	1980		1985		Change (1980–85)	
	n	Per cent	n	Per cent	n	Per cent
Senior Nurse Grade 7 or Equivalent*	32.0	2.0	116.0	4.2	84.0	262.5
Senior Nurse Grade 8 or Equivalent**	147.0	8.8	65.0	2.4	−82.0	−55.0
Charge Nurse 1	58.5	3.5	86.0	3.1	27.5	47.0
Charge Nurse 2	1144.0	68.5	2084.0	76.0	940.0	82.0
Staff Nurse	137.5	8.2	206.0	7.4	68.5	50.0
State Enrolled Nurse	130.5	7.8	163.0	6.0	32.5	25.0
Nursing Assistant	17.5	1.2	12.0	0.9	−5.5	−31.5
TOTAL	1667.0	100.0	2758.0	100.0	1091.0	65.5

*Includes Nursing Officer 1 and Senior Nursing Officer.
**Includes Nursing Officer 2.

Source: CPNA Surveys 1980 and 1985.

this level. However, the increase in the numbers employed on the Senior Nurse grade 7 scale almost exactly mirrors the decline in the use of the Nursing Officer banding.

At a managerial level, then, most CPN services, and certainly those in England and Wales, are now spearheaded by a Senior Nurse grade 7, whereas in 1980 the service manager was most likely to be a Nursing Officer (grade 2). The most common management arrangement in England and Wales is for a Senior Nurse, grade 7 or 8, to report directly to a Director of Nursing Services (this occurs in 70% of all CPN teams in the United Kingdom). In Scotland and Northern Ireland, the most usual system is for a Nursing Officer to report directly to an intermediate Senior Nursing Officer. The 1982 National Health Service reorganisation accounts for this difference. In England and Wales the reorganisation coincided with the introduction of a new senior nurse structure which it did not in the other countries.

There has been a very small increase in the use of the Charge Nurse, grade 1 post (27.5 whole time equivalents (WTE)). Twelve of these posts have been created in one district in Wales, where completion of ENB cc no. 810 (in community psychiatric nursing) warrants automatic promotion to this level. However, since 1980 a minimum of 940 new Charge Nurse grade 2 posts have been established nationally and there are now over 2000 CPNs employed at this grade.

Specialist CPNs

The strong growth of the total CPN workforce is paralleled by the numbers of CPNs who now work in an exclusive specialty. The 1980 CPNA survey found that 62 services (28%) offered a specialist service in addition to general psychiatry. The 1985 survey investigated the question of specialism in a different way, looking at the number of CPNs within services who worked exclusively with one client group. The results show that the largest area of specialist work for CPNs is with the elderly (see Table 3.2). Throughout the country, one in five CPNs are working with this group of people. Overall the astonishingly high

Table 3.2   NATIONAL BREAKDOWN OF CPNS BY SPECIALISM

Specialism	n	Per cent
Elderly	505	64.0
Crisis work	100	12.6
Drugs/alcohol	72	9.0
Rehabilitation	42	5.2
Children	36	4.5
Behaviour therapy	36	4.5
Family therapy	2	0.2
TOTAL	793	100.0

Source: CPNA Survey 1985.

figure of 29% of all CPNs are working exclusively with one client group.

CPN growth: an explanation

CPN specialisation appears to have been a major factor in the increase in the CPN workforce. But what other factors have been important? CPNs themselves, intuitively and subjectively, place a high value on the work they do, but they undoubtedly share this outlook in common with other professional groups! This alone cannot have been enough to convince high-level policy-makers and planners that such a rapid expansion in CPN services was vital. Indeed only a few years ago CPNs were warned that future growth in services was only likely if they could prove their clinical efficiency through research (Mangen and Griffith, 1982). So how have these great increases in CPNs come about?

The concentration of CPNs varies across the UK. This is shown in Table 3.3 which breaks down the average CPN team size within RHAs and countries for the years 1980 and 1985. In Scotland, for example, the average CPN team size was 6.8 WTEs in 1985, comparing unfavourably with, say, the South-western RHA in England which had average team sizes of 17.6 CPNs for the same period. Regional inequalities in health care exist and have been well documented, and the work of the Resource Allocation Working Party (RAWP) has attempted to redistribute NHS finance to rectify these imbalances (see Chapter 2). In the area of CPN provision, RAWP appears to have been relatively successful. RHAs such as Trent, East Anglia and Wessex, all large RAWP-receiving areas, had large increases in CPN personnel, with average increases in CPN workforces per team of 9.3, 8.9 and 7.7 respectively. However, the RAWP policy alone is not enough to explain the large CPN team increases – other factors have been at play.

Some small scale research highlights these factors (Brooker, 1985). First, Directors of Nursing Services seem to have been adept at exploiting the various possible sources of funding for new CPN posts. These include regional development monies (that is, "pump priming"), transfers from existing nursing budgets, joint finance, district development money, EEC inner-city aid programmes and central DHSS sources, particularly for drug and alcohol specialist CPN posts.

The second factor, again, appears to be hospital closures. In the majority of the health authorities examined, further increases in CPN personnel were being predicted, all linked with plans to close the large psychiatric hospitals. For example, one health authority in the Wessex RHA plans to open four community mental health centres each served by eight CPNs, a development approved only if the psychiatric hospital in the DHA reduced its beds by 50% over the next seven years. Similarly, a DHA in East Anglia is

Table 3.3   AVERAGE CPN TEAM SIZE

RHA/Country	Size (1980)	Size (1985)	Net change
Yorkshire	3.8	8.9	+5.1
Northern	5.8	9.0	+3.2
Trent	5.9	15.2	+9.3
East Anglia	4.6	13.5	+8.9
North-west Thames	6.6	13.1	+6.5
North-east Thames	8.2	13.5	+5.3
South-east Thames	7.8	12.6	+4.8
South-west Thames	9.5	14.2	+4.7
Wessex	9.0	16.7	+7.7
Oxford	10.2	14.5	+4.3
South-western	8.3	17.6	+9.3
West Midlands	7.0	12.2	+5.2
Mersey	6.6	12.1	+5.5
North-western	7.1	11.3	+4.2
Wales	—	16.7	—
Scotland	—	6.8	—
Northern Ireland	—	8.0	—
Mean	7.0	12.7	+5.7

Source: CPNA Surveys 1980 and 1985

planning to close a 600-bed hospital entirely in 1994, and the CPN team will increase from 17 to 40 over this time-span to allow for community support of the transferred patients. Of course, not all DHAs have firm hospital closure policies; this is particularly so in Scotland. But where such policies do exist, CPN team growth will be correspondingly significant.

Third, the research showed that local relationships with other professional colleagues are important in creating a climate within which CPN teams can expand. In areas where CPN services are well established and have demonstrated their viability, psychiatrists have become firm advocates for them. This is particularly true in specialisms where psychiatrists are keen that CPNs mirror their own organisational practices. In DHAs where CPNs have demonstrated their usefulness to general practitioners, the latter have been convinced very swiftly of the value of CPN attachments. Relationships with local authorities are also very important for CPNs, particularly as "joint finance" can fund new jobs. However, major difficulties still exist in many DHAs because of the role overlap between CPNs and social workers. This issue is examined in more depth in Chapter 6.

In summary, the size of a CPN team is inextricably linked with what it is trying to achieve. Whether or not it can expand to achieve those aims depends on:

- Workforce levels – that is, given local funding availability how many nurses can be realistically expected to be deployed?
- Local relationships with consultant psychiatrists and GPs – is the referral system open or closed?
- Local relationships with other nursing colleagues, such as district nurses and health visitors.
- The style of local general management.
- The size and type of DHA. Is it predominantly urban or rural? What size population does it serve?
- The level of postbasic clinical skills acquired by individual nurses within the team and subsequently their degree of clinical specialism.
- Whether or not there is a local policy to run down and close the nearest large psychiatric hospital.
- The relationship with the local authority and consequent use of joint finance.
- Crucially, where the team members themselves are to be located.
- The nature of the nursing philosophy that underpins the individual CPN service.

Finally, and perhaps of over-riding significance, is the ability of individual CPN service managers to articulate the appropriateness of these factors in planning the future direction and expansion of the team.

Formal CPN workforce planning ratio

Formal CPN workforce planning ratios are formulas which determine the need to have one CPN per proportion of the DHA population. The commonest appears to be the recommendation that nationally there should be one CPN per 10 000 people in the population.

The history and origin of CPN workforce ratios is interesting and comes from research carried out in the Chester region in the 1970s. Driver (1976) established from a sample of GPs that they would refer 13.13% of their patients with mental health problems to a CPN, if available. Carr, Butterworth and Hodges (1980) use this figure of 13.13% in the following way:

● They estimate that the number of patients consulting their GP with mental health problems per year is 140 per 1000 (this figure draws on the work of Shepherd *et al.*, 1966).

● Thus, if one CPN was available per 15 000 of the population there would be a potential pool of 2100 people with mental health problems (that is, $140 \times 15 = 2100$).

● Driver's work estimates that of these 2100 people, GPs would like to refer 13.13% (or 276 clients) to CPNs.

● Thus if there were one CPN per 7500 of the population, GPs would refer 138 new clients to CPNs per year.

This then is the calculation upon which Carr and his colleagues recommend the ratio of one CPN per 15 000 of the population, a figure the CPNA revised downwards to one CPN per 7500 of the population.

There are, however, many dangers in adopting such a formula in a wholesale manner. First, as Driver (1976, p. 100) points out: "If a similar piece of research of the same magnitude was carried out in the same place . . . an entirely different set of statistics may be produced." Or in other words, the way GPs perceive the demand for CPN services will vary, as will the incidence of mental health problems in each DHA's population. Also, if we accept the theory that the ratio 1:15 000 means that 276 new clients are referred each year, this implies that CPNs are accepting referrals from GPs only, which is patently not the case.

It is also difficult to understand what exactly the figure of 276 clients per year means. How often would each of these people need to be seen? What are their problems? Just how does the number relate to the actual working practices of a GP-attached CPN?

Although many difficulties are associated with formal workforce planning targets, many RHAs have adopted them. Wessex and East Anglia RHAs, for example, suggest that DHAs should be working towards population ratios of one CPN per 10 000 population. Table 3.4 shows the progress of RHAs in achieving such targets. Overall there has been an outstanding improvement from a ratio of one CPN per 50 000 in 1980 to one CPN per 21.000 in 1985, the most dramatic improvements being in the South-east Thames and East Anglia RHAs.

Table 3.4   REGIONAL POPULATION RATIOS PER CPN IN ENGLAND
(1980 AND 1985)

Region	Rank	Ratio (1980)	Rank	Ratio (1985)	1980–85 Ratio
North-east Thames	1	31 700	4	19 000	1.67
North-western	2	37 400	9	22 300	1.68
South-western	3	37 800	2	18 000	2.10
Wessex	4	38 300	1	17 800	2.15
South-west Thames	5	38 600	6	21 250	1.82
Oxford	6	39 500	7	21 300	1.85
West Midlands	7	42 000	9	22 300	1.88
Mersey	8	42 300	12	24 200	1.75
Northern	9	53 300	7	21 300	2.50
North-west Thames	10	58 900	11	22 800	2.58
South-east Thames	11	60 000	3	18 130	3.31
Trent	12	72 400	13	27 150	2.67
East Anglia	13	74 000	5	20 000	3.70
Yorkshire	14	75 200	14	34 500	2.18
Total		50 000		21 000	2.10

Source: CPNA Surveys 1980 and 1985.

If the ratio recommendation of 1:10 000 were applied to all CPN teams then on average district CPN teams would vary between 20 and 45 CPNs per team (See Fig. 3.2). This target, while very healthy in terms of absolute numbers, is not based on any local assessment of need. So we must summarise here with a plea: the future planning of CPN services must not occur using the "top-down" approach recently adopted by some RHAs; we must rid ourselves of the idea that we need so many CPNs per head of the population. Individual CPNs and their managers have a responsibility, well described by Rae (1985):

To take the initiative in their own districts, and ensure that, along with their colleagues, operational plans are composed that will meet the individual needs of clients. If we fail to confront those issues and do not respond positively, we will be judged as accomplices to the serious decline of psychiatric nursing, guilty of neglecting to protect the future interests of mentally disabled people.

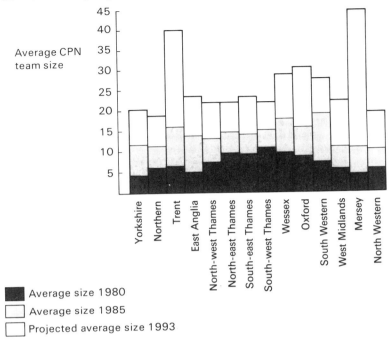

Fig. 3.2   Average CPN team size by region.

Base and referral pattern

CPN base

There is, of course, no "typical" CPN service – hopefully the style of CPN service offered relates to the locally assessed demand for community-oriented psychiatric nursing care. However, there is a clear link between where and how CPNs work and the source of their referrals. The role for a CPN based in a large hospital receiving all referrals from a psychiatrist is fundamentally different to that of, say, the CPN, based in a health clinic, accepting the majority of referrals from a GP. On the one hand, the hospital CPN will be involved in tertiary prevention, following-up and providing after-care for discharged psychiatric patients. On the other hand, the health clinic CPN is more likely to be concerned with secondary prevention, in other words, decreasing the likelihood of admission for clients in the first place.

In 1980 77% of all CPNs were based either in a psychiatric hospital or psychiatric units in District General Hospitals (DGHs)

(Table 3.5). By 1985 this had changed with 20% fewer CPNs using hospitals as a main work setting. Nevertheless the largest group of CPNs (37.35% or 962 CPNs) still work out of psychiatric hospitals, and 56.45% work out of psychiatric hospitals or psychiatric units in DGHs.

Table 3.5 CPNS BY MAIN BASE (1980 AND 1985)

	1980 Per cent	1985 Per cent	1985 n	Change (Per cent)
Psychiatric hospital	49.0	37.35	962	−11.65
Psychiatric unit (DGH)	28.0	19.1	492	−8.9
Health Centre/General practitioner practice	8.0	17.15	442	+9.15
Day hospital	8.0	9.8	252	+1.8
Mental health centre (other)	7.0	16.2	427	+9.6
Total	100.0	100.0	2575*	0.0

*This figure differs from the total figure in Table 3.1, as service managers are not included.

There is considerable regional variation in this pattern however. Table 3.6 shows that in the North-western RHA, CPNs are most likely to be found in the psychiatric unit of a DGH, whereas in Northern Ireland and the South-east Thames RHA, CPNs work overwhelmingly from health centres or GP practices. In Scotland, very nearly seven in ten CPNs are based in psychiatric hospitals, whereas in the North-western region only two CPNs in ten are likely to be based in such a setting.

The relationship between referral and base

So how does the base of CPNs affect their referral pattern, caseload and ultimately their role? What is the evidence to suggest that such an equation exists? If we look at the way in which medical referrals to CPNs vary by region and country (Table 3.7), we can begin to understand this interplay.

Scottish CPNs are most likely to be based in psychiatric hospitals, and as a result they receive more referrals from psychiatrists than anywhere else in the country (see Table 3.7). Alternatively CPNs in South-east Thames were among those most likely to be located in primary care, and as a group they obtained fewest referrals from psychiatrists. This is not a watertight case, however; for example, CPNs in the South-western RHA are more

Table 3.6 PERCENTAGE OF CPN WORKFORCE BY AREA AND BASE

RHA/Country	Psychiatric hospital	DGH unit	Health centre/general practitioner practice	Day hospital	Other
Yorkshire	27.0	33.0	1.5*	18.0	20.5
Northern	47.7	14.4	17.5	8.3	12.1
Trent	39.0	6.6	23.7	9.7	21.0
East Anglia	63.0	9.9	12.3	8.7	6.1
North-west Thames	29.3	36.4	12.0	1.6*	20.7
North-east Thames	39.2	12.0	33.5	5.1	10.2
South-east Thames	14.8*	16.5	33.7	7.0	28.0
South-west Thames	33.5	20.5	25.4	7.1	13.5
Wessex	45.5	11.4	4.1	18.0	21.0
Oxford	40.5	8.6	3.4	17.4	30.1**
South-western	44.3	16.5	3.1	19.1**	17.0
West Midlands	36.0	15.2	15.6	9.7	23.5
Mersey	60.2	32.9	2.4	2.5	2.0*
North-western	17.2	48.2**	18.6	2.3	13.7
Wales	36.8	7.7	38.3	11.2	6.0
Scotland	69.5**	6.0	11.6	6.2	6.7
Northern Ireland	33.9	3.2*	43.5**	3.2	16.1

*Lowest in range.
**Highest in range.

Table 3.7 UNITED KINGDOM VARIATION IN MEDICAL REFERRALS (MEAN PER CENT)

RHA/Country	Referral source (per cent)	
	Psychiatrist	General practitioner
Yorkshire	73.5	14.3
North	50.27	35.5
Trent	56.56	28.8
East Anglia	54.2	19.7
North-west Thames	66.5	20.3
North-east Thames	46.3	27.8
South-east Thames	41.5*	29.14
South-west Thames	47.6	24.75
Wessex	70.0	10.5*
Oxford	66.6	25.4
South-western	46.9	43.2**
West Midlands	58.6	23.8
Mersey	62.7	12.3
North-western	52.7	26.28
Wales	66.9	24.3
Scotland	81.9**	13.8
Northern Ireland	51.3	22.4
Total	59.35	23.27

*Lowest in range.
**Highest in range.

commonly found in day hospitals yet receive more referrals from GPs. But in general these results point up a consistent trend.

At the end of the 1970s, the era of experimentation for CPNs, there was an understandable ambivalence about the best place to locate CPN services. This has been summarised by Carr, Butterworth and Hodges (1980): "From the inception of CPN services there has been considerable discussion as to the most suitable site for the service. Should teams be based in hospital, community or health centres, or a mixture of the three?" Whether CPNs should see discharged hospital patients as a priority or consider the needs of clients in primary health care, is still under debate (Community Nursing Review Team, 1985). In considering the experimental attachment of CPNs to general practice in Oxford, Leopoldt and Hurn's (1973) answer to the problem was a compromise. They believed that CPNs should divide their time equally between GPs and psychiatrists, and added: "As long as the psychiatric hospital remains in the centre of the specialist service, it is desirable for CPNs to remain hospital based and a member of the specialist team."

However, the opposite has also been argued. Community nurses working from hospitals may find it very difficult to avoid being heavily influenced by the medical model (Campbell, Dixon and Dow, 1983). There are also other advantages that can accrue to CPNs working from community bases: liaison is facilitated with other community workers, there may be new clinical fields in which to gain experience, and (more prosaically) travelling distance and time is reduced.

The House of Commons Social Services Select Committee Report (1985) made it very clear that they felt that it was inappropriate for CPN teams to operate "closed" referral systems, saying to the Royal College of Psychiatrists that:

> We would welcome a statement from the RCP specifically encouraging the idea of a direct referral from GP to CPNs. If that is not to inhibit a CPN's role in providing for discharged hospital patients, some expansion of the CPN Service will be required (para 194).

There is reason to worry, however, that as CPNs move to community bases, patients with chronic mental illness will receive less of their attention. Goldberg (1985), examining mental health in Lancashire, argues that the build-up of CPN services has been a key factor in reducing the average length of stay of patients admitted to the psychiatric unit of a teaching DGH, the mean length of stay being reduced from 42.5 days in 1974 to 28.6 days in 1982. However, he is not happy about the CPN move to primary care settings. He suggests (1985, p. 60)

> that the effect of the move to primary care is a great increase in unsupervised work with patients with depression and other neuroses who have not been seen by secondary care services . . . as CPNs drift away from the hospital based service there is a risk that care of the chronic psychotic patients will take second place to work with people with minor affective disorders.

Goldberg is right to stress the importance of community work with the chronic mentally ill, and this is of particular importance in those districts currently pursuing active hospital closure programmes.

There is, therefore, a range of opinions about CPN service organisation, and these opinions come from a cross-section of mental health care professionals. Is there evidence to suggest that it actually matters where a CPN is based?

Williamson, Little and Lindsay (1981) evaluated two CPN

teams: one operating from a hospital (team A) and one based in a health centre (team B). Team B received referrals from a wider range of sources, was able to follow-up specialist referrals, and carried out a greater number of visits. Patients expressed equal satisfaction with both services. (Lebow (1982) has shown, however, that dissatisfied clients do not stay in treatment so such a finding may not tell us a great deal.)

Skidmore and Friend (1984) interviewed 120 CPNs from 12 CPN services chosen at random throughout the country and found some differences and some similarities between CPNs by bases. CPNs in primary health care were referred the same number of "new" cases as CPNs who were hospital-based, and CPNs in both settings spent the same amount of time with clients and relatives; 83% of the CPNs themselves were in favour of bases in both settings. An example of this attitude was: "There is a lot that can be done in primary care but CPN services need the backing of the hospital." There were, however, significant differences in the source of referral depending on CPN base. The primary health care-based CPN received far more referrals from non-medical sources than did the hospital-based CPN – 42% compared with 13% – and self-referrals of new clients were five times more likely for the primary health care-based CPN than for his or her hospital-based colleague. Hospital-based CPNs appeared to be more directed by doctors in their ultimate intervention, while primary health care CPNs appeared to enjoy more autonomy in deciding how to deal with referrals. Skidmore and Friend conclude their article by asserting that there is a necessary role for CPNs in primary health care, but they also recommend that CPN teams investigate local referral sources so as to understand the factors that precipitate the referrals *before* the decision is taken as to where CPNs should be deployed.

This was very much the thinking behind a study we carried out to examine the effect of "base" on referrals and CPN caseload activity in an Inner London Health District (Brooker and Simmons, 1985). In this DHA, part of the CPN team (4) was based in a day hospital and the remainder (5) in health clinics. We wanted to know whether there is a difference in the type of client referred to the two "teams", and also whether there are differences in aspects of CPN activity, such as number of referrals, caseload size and where sessions actually took place.

The results indicated that clients referred to the day hospital-based team were more likely to be aged between 16–30, male and single, whereas the health centre team's clients were predominantly married, female and aged 31–45 (see Table 3.8). In addition day hospital clients were more likely to live in hostels and bed and breakfasts, while health centre clients were mostly in rented accommodation.

The largest single group of referrers to both teams were general practitioners. The teams did deal with different client groups, and this is largely a reflection of the local population's need and the subsequent organisation of the two teams. Finally, we demonstrated that day hospital-based CPNs spend a significantly smaller proportion of their time in clinical contact with clients than their health centre colleagues. This is probably because they spend more time travelling to clients.

This research has had a significant local impact, and since its publication the overall service has been expanded and a new team created, attached to primary health care and made up of a number of the former day hospital CPNs. Many CPNs who orient themselves to the community worry that links with psychiatric hospitals and out-patient departments will be weakened. Interestingly, our study suggested the referrals from psychiatrists and ward-based staff were higher in the health clinic-attached team than the one based in the day hospital.

Summary

CPN team organisation is changing. CPN staffing levels increased dramatically between 1980 and 1985, and it is possible that the current national CPN workforce of some 3000 may rise to 8000 if regional manpower planning targets are implemented. These vast manpower increases are, in many cases, linked with large psychiatric hospital closures. CPN service managers should base their estimation of CPN staffing requirements on an assessment of local need, and not simply use formulas such as one CPN per 10 000 of the population.

We close this chapter with a reminder. This book examines the idea that CPNs' clients are part of a system, and it proposes a model of community psychiatric nursing that is essentially psychosocial. Many CPNs see a move from hospital to community setting as an escape from "the prevailing medical ideology". Hopefully, the subsequent chapters will enable the CPN to

Table 3.8 REFERRING AGENT BY CPN BASE

Referrer	Day hospital-based		Health-clinic based		Total	
	n	Per cent	n	Per cent	n	Per cent
General practitioner	39	39.8	32	43.2	71	41.3
Social worker	6	6.1	4	5.4	10	5.8
Community nurses	7	7.1	10	13.5	17	9.9
Psychiatrists and hospital	9	9.2	13	17.6	22	12.8
Hostel	0	0	7	9.5	7	4.1
Age Concern	2	2.0	1	1.4	3	1.7
Day centre	2	2.0	0	0	2	1.2
Day hospital	4	4.1	2	2.7	6	3.5
WECVS*	24	24.5	0	0	24	14.5
Self	1	1.0	3	4.1	4	2.3
Other	4	4.1	2	2.7	6	3.5
Total	98	57.0	74	43.0	172	100.0

*West End Coordinated Voluntary Services.

Source: Brooker and Simmons [1985].

determine a model of nursing care in the community which has a sound philosophical and theoretical foundation.

References

Aire, T. and Isaacs, D. (1978) The development of psychiatric services for the elderly in Britain, in *Studies in Generic Psychiatry* (eds A. D. Isaacs and F. Post). John Wiley, New York.

Baxter, Y. (1984) Conference Opening Remarks, *Community Psychiatric Nursing Journal*, **4**(3), 11.

Brooker, C. (1985) *The 1985 National Community Psychiatric Nursing Survey Update: Implications of the findings for the evolution of a survey methodology.* Unpublished MSc thesis, City University.

Brooker, C. and Simmons, S. (1985) A study to compare two models of community psychiatric nursing care delivery. *Journal of Advanced Nursing*, **10**, 217–23.

Brooker, C. and Brown, M. (1986) National follow up survey of practising nurse therapists, in *Readings in Psychiatric Nursing Research* (ed. J. Brooking), Chapter 10, Wiley and Sons, Chichester.

Campbell, W., Dixon, A. and Dow I. (1983) A case for a new training. *Nursing Mirror*, **156**, 42–6.

Carr, P., Butterworth, C. A. and Hodges, B. E. (1980) *Community Psychiatric Nursing*, Churchill-Livingstone, Edinburgh.

Community Psychiatric Nurses Association (1980) *National Survey of Community Psychiatric Nursing Services.* CPNA Publications, Leeds.

Community Psychiatric Nurses Association (1985) *The 1985 CPNA National Survey Update.* CPNA Publications, Leeds.

Corser, C. and Ryce, S. (1977) Community mental health care: A model based on the primary health care system. *British medical Journal*, **2**, 936–8.

Delay and Deniker (1952) *In* Lader, M. (1976) *The history of pharmacology.* Smith, Kline and French, England.

Driver, E. (1976). *Assessment of the demand for a CPN service in Chester.* CPN Research monographs No. 1, Manchester Polytechnic.

Goldberg, D. (1985). *Mental Health Policies in Lancashire.* Presented at joint DHSS/Royal College of Psychiatrists Conference on community care.

Griffith, J. H. and Mangen, S. P. (1980). Community psychiatric nursing – a literature review. *International Journal of Nursing Studies*, **17**, 197–210.

Health Advisory Service (1982) The rising tide.

Henderson, J. (1945) *Modern Mental Nursing*, Vol. 3, Caxton.

Her Majesty's Stationery Office (1979) Royal Commission on the National Health Service.

House of Commons, Social Service Select Committee Report (1985). Community care: with special reference to adult mentally ill and mentally handicapped people. *House of Commons Paper 13,1*, vol.1. HMSO, London.

Hunter, P. (1974) Community psychiatric nursing in Britain: an historical review. *International Journal of Nursing Studies*, **11**.

Lebow, J. (1982) Consumer satisfaction with mental health treatment. *Psychological Bulletin*, **91**(2), 244–59.

Leopoldt, H. and Hurn, R. (1973) Towards integration. *Nursing Mirror*, **136**, 38–42.

Mangen, S. P. and Griffith, J. H. (1982) CPN Services in Britain: the need for policy and planning. *International Journal of Nursing Studies*, **19**(3), 157–65.

May, A. R. and Moore, S. (1963) The mental nurse in the community. *Lancet*, **1**, 213–14.

McKendrick, D. (1980) *Statistical returns in community psychiatric nursing*, unpublished project, Manchester Polytechnic.

Nursing Times (1985) Editorial. **81**, (10), 30.

Parnell, J. W. (1978) *Community psychiatric nursing: a descriptive study*. Queen's Nursing Institute, London.

Paykel, E. S. and Griffith, J. H. (1983) *Community Psychiatric Nursing for Neurotic Patients*. RCN, London.

Peat, L. and Watt, G. (1984) The passing of an era. *Community Psychiatric Nursing Journal*, **4**, (2), 12–16.

Peplau, H. (1952) *Interpersonal relations in nursing*. Putnam, New York.

Rae, M. (1985) No ostriches please. *Senior Nurse*, **3**(3), 10.

Royal College of Nursing (1966) *Investigation into the role of the psychiatric nurse in the community*. Unpublished.

Royal College of Psychiatrists (1980) Community psychiatric nursing – a discussion document. *Bulletin of the Royal College of Psychiatrists*, **August**, 117–21.

Royal Medico-Psychological Association (1969) Report of the committee on local authorities and allied personal social services. Royal Medico-Psychological Association, London.

Shepherd, M., Cooper, B., Brown, A. C., and Kalton, G. (1966). *Psychiatric Illness in General Practice*. Oxford University Press, London.

Shore, A. (1977) *An appraisal of the existing CPN services in the North Western Region*. CPN Research monograph No. 19, Manchester Polytechnic.

Skidmore, D. and Friend, W. (1985) Should CPNs be in the primary health care team? *Nursing Times, Community Outlook*, **9 September**, 310–12.

Strobie, E. G. and Hopkins, D. H. (1972) Crisis intervention. A psychiatric community nurse in a rural area. *Nursing Times*, **68**, 165–8.

Tooth, G. C. and Brook, E. (1961) Trends in the mental health population and their effect on planning. *Lancet*, **1 April**, 710–13.

Williamson, F., Little, M. and Lindsay, W. (1981) Two CPN services compared. *Nursing Times*, **77**, 105–7.

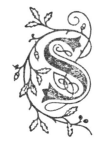

4

The Individual, the Family and the CPN

The Family, the Individual and Mental Health

Community psychiatric nurses are concerned with people's mental health. But what do we mean by mental health? Is it simply an absence of mental illness, or is it, as the World Health Organisation's famous definition suggests, a "state of positive well-being"? Dubos is quoted as saying "health is not a state of being: it is a process of adaptation to the changing demands of living and the changing meanings we give to life itself" (Robinson, 1971). In other words health, including mental health, cannot be defined in any fixed or absolute sense, but must be understood as dependent on variable social, cultural and family factors. However, Clare has outlined the dangers of adopting a definition of mental health based exclusively on a set of social values. He suggests (Clare, 1976, p. 15) that if this were the case we would say:

> The mentally healthy person is not a nuisance, does not challenge the rules, lose his temper, kick the cat, or park his car on a double yellow line. He makes no demands, passes his life quietly and productively and does not fiddle the social security, live with a mistress, or wear placards warning that the end of the world is nigh.

This does not mean that we can go no further. Indeed, many writers have attempted to describe a set of prerequisites for psychological equilibrium or mental health. One such list includes: love, support, impulse control, feeling part of a group, and personal achievement and recognition (Caplan, 1969). Many of these are initially found or learned in the family group; others, particularly the last two, may be more often gained through work or other occupational activity, and social participation outside of the family. Maslow (1968) has devised a much more complex model of needs or motivations (that is, something which incites action, or which sustains or gives direction to an action) which he arranges into a hierarchy (Fig. 4.1).

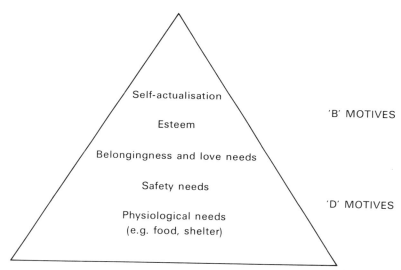

Fig. 4.1 Maslow's hierarchy

The lower needs are described as "deficiency" motives, those that are triggered by a lack of something. The higher "being" motives can only come into play once the lower level needs of survival and safety have been addressed. The highest motivating drive is that of self-actualisation, described by Maslow as the process of developing one's potential to the full, and recognisable from a cluster of characteristics including: efficient perception of reality and comfortable relations with it, acceptance of self and others, spontaneity, sense of humour, creativeness and individuality.

Another of the higher level needs in this model is that of esteem. This refers to both the esteem of others and self-esteem. The latter is often described as low in those who seek psychiatric help or counselling. Self-esteem is closely linked to self-confidence, assertiveness, the feeling that alternatives exist in one's life, and that one can cope ·-ith most problems that may arise. Clearly,

Maslow's "B" motives and belongingness, esteem (from self and others) and self-actualisation are closely related to Caplan's list of requirements for mental health. This would suggest, therefore, that true mental health (in the sense of more than the mere absence of illness) requires that basic needs are met. An individual's needs for esteem and self-actualisation are of course less pressing than, and therefore give way to, needs for shelter, food, etc. Many of those receiving psychiatric treatment come from the poorer and disadvantaged sections of society, who often have many associated problems of low income, poor housing and unemployment. While these problems remain unsolved, will positive mental health be a realistic goal for them? In the day-to-day work of CPNs this may mean that some clients require help with such important areas of their lives as housing. In some cases CPNs will be able to give relevant advice or information, but in other instances they may refer the client to colleagues in the social services or housing departments.

Where then does a person get the ideas, attitudes to mental health, orientations and, in some cases, skills that will accompany him or her through life? These, and in addition ideas concerning life goals and expectations and opportunities and ability to address higher level needs, are all to some extent learned and reinforced within the family and other primary groups, including school, peer group and, later, occupational group. Such a group is not simply a conglomeration of individuals, but has an identity, a history and a culture of its own. These groups can be described as systems, and their characteristics can be examined and discussed by using general systems theory. The family is the most important of these.

The family system

The term "system" is one borrowed originally from the physical sciences. It has been defined as a "set of objects together with the relationships between the objects and between their attributes. The objects are the component parts of the system, the attributes are the properties of the objects and the relationships tie the system together" (Hall and Fagen, quoted in Walrond-Skinner, 1977). When this definition is applied to the most commonly occurring social system – the family – it becomes clear that the objects of the system are the family members, their attributes are the members' characteristics and the relationships become the relationships between the family members, in this case binding the family system together.

A system, then, is more than the sum of its parts. It becomes a whole within which its component parts (the family members) can only be understood as parts of the whole. Taking the mechanical analogy of a car engine we can see that a breakdown in one element of the system, say the ignition timing, will affect all other components, and may lead to the whole system becoming inoperative. Likewise within a family, change in one of the members will affect the lives of all other members of that family. This is particularly marked when, for example, a new baby joins the family causing all other family members to make major adjustments. Similarly, family systems change greatly when the main breadwinner becomes unemployed.

In science, systems may be described as "open" or "closed", depending on whether there is communication between the system and the wider environment. In social systems such as families there could not, of course, be any such thing as a totally closed system. Families depend on their relationships with others for their survival. These external relationships form the family's network – made up of relatives, friends, work colleagues, and other groups with whom the family has regular contact. If many of the members of the network also relate to each other independently of the central family, the network can be described as "highly connected". If, on the other hand, there are few other relationships among the network it is considered to be "dispersed". This is illustrated in Fig. 4.2.

Although it is not possible to exist as a completely closed family system, it is possible to consider families as being relatively open or relatively closed, depending on the degree of communication across the boundary between the family, their network and the wider community. An open family system engages in a considerable amount of communication with its suprasystem (network) and also among its subsystems – individual members and groupings. In contrast, a relatively closed family system appears to have limited interchange between family members or with the wider network. In such families there is simply less communication or exchange going on at any level.

Walrond-Skinner (1977) makes the point that we cannot simply assume that open families are functional or healthy, while closed families are neither. She points out that Minuchin has used a similar way of dividing families into two broad types –

Highly connected   Dispersed

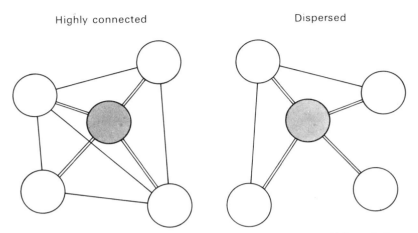

Fig. 4.2   Highly connected and dispersed family systems. (Adpated from Anderson, 1971)

"disengaged" and "enmeshed" – which relate in part to the open–closed division. Disengaged families are those in which there is little communication among members, while enmeshed families tend to have a high level of involvement. To illustrate, if a CPN were to suggest family meetings to a disengaged family he or she might find that these meetings were the only time that the family communicated together at all. At the other extreme, many CPNs will be familiar with families in which family members appear very involved with each other, and individual growth and developing independence are hindered. In such enmeshed families the CPN's work might aim to help reduce the family's over-involvement and allow individual members to become somewhat more separate.

To take the scientific analogy a stage further, the concept of "homeostasis" has been used. In physical sciences this refers to the mechanism within a system whereby information about changes in one part of the system is fed back to another section so that the operation of the second part is adjusted accordingly. The most commonly used example (and we can find no better) is that of the domestic central heating system with its in-built thermostat. The thermostat monitors the temperature of a certain part of the house, and on the basis of this information "instructs" the boiler when to start up or close down. When the temperature drops below a certain point the boiler comes on, only to stop when the thermostat registers a particular higher temperature. In this way the temperature of the house is kept within fairly narrow limits and the occupants stay comfortable. Families also develop mechanisms which may be used to maintain a balance, a status quo, within them. Many CPNs will have experienced, either in their own families (where it is often more difficult to recognise), or in the families of their clients, the predictable argument that always ends in the same way, or the child who always cries at the same moment of tension in a conflict between her parents.

A degree of homeostasis within a family – the capacity to remain constant in spite of changing external conditions – is of course very important. The members of a family require and will seek some stability, some constancies, within the family system, when there may be great changes happening in other parts of their lives, such as at school or at work. However, it would be wrong to take the concept too far, since over-rigid homeostatic mechanisms within the family may prevent any growth occurring among members and in the family as a whole. It seems that the ideal family (were it to exist) would strike a healthy balance between providing stability and security for all its members and, at different stages of their development, helping members to grow, take on new roles, and when appropriate, leave the family home. Sometimes the intervention of a CPN, by supporting a particular family member, could help to maintain a precarious family homeostasis. This may often be beneficial, but at other times the CPN's action may be preventing movement within the family needed for growth. Clearly, as with the concept of the closed system, the total adoption of the scientific model of homeostasis would be inappropriate. However, we may still take something from it.

We pointed out earlier that no individual family system may exist without there being some communication with the wider society, sometimes referred to as the suprasystem. Just as the family is one unit in this larger suprasystem, the family system itself may be broken down into subsystems (Caplan, 1969).

The first subsystem is the marital system, which is generally a "close" one, in the sense of being intimate. In some families, however, the marital relationship may never be close, possibly because one partner has not been able to truly leave his or her family of origin (that is, the family in which a person has grown up). In Chapter 2 we discussed Young and Wilmott's different types of family organisation. In their stage 2 families the close and continuing bond between a mother and her married daughter is much stronger than that of husband and wife. It has been suggested that if a young woman goes straight from the home of her family of origin to her marital home, she spends no time as an unattached young adult, which is often an important stage in separation from parents in western society. Where a very close relationship does exist between family members it may, on occasion, develop into an alliance formed in opposition to others – for example, a women's alliance against their male family members, or a mother and son's alliance against the son's wife.

If a close marital subsystem does exist, when children enter the family it must become less close in order to allow the parent–child relationships or sub-systems to develop. If there is some ambivalence in the parents towards the new baby they may be less willing to give "space" to him or her, wishing to hang on to their cosy partnership; or there may be resentment or rivalry between one parent and the child for the attention of the other parent.

When the marital relationship is not close the arrival of a child can lead to one or other of the parents becoming particularly involved with the child or children. This can then disguise a rather empty marital relationship from which the husband and wife receive little support. By putting their energies into their children, they put off the need to examine or challenge their own relationship. Later, when the time comes for the children to leave the family home, the original marital subsystem becomes central once again. At this point there is a need for this system to become close again. If this does not happen and the relationship remains somewhat distant or acrimonious, the child may have difficulty in leaving home, or there may be a tendency for one or other of the partners (more often the mother as we have seen) to follow the son or daughter out and into their new home. Clearly, this has an effect on the new family system being established by the young person, and he or she may, as a consequence, have difficulty forming a close marital relationship. We are thus back at our starting point, having come full circle.

The notion that we can think about families moving in a circular rather than a simple linear way is one that has been considered and elaborated by others (see, for example, Haley, 1973; Carter and McGoldrick, 1980). Such writers suggest that families go through a series of developmental stages just as individuals do, and that each stage imposes a series of tasks. Just as individuals may have difficulty in getting past a certain stage, so too may families. Six stages are commonly identified, although they may overlap at times (Table 4.1).

Table 4.1 FAMILY LIFE-CYCLE (adapted from Haley (1973) and Carter and McGoldrick (1980))

Stage	Tasks facing the family and changes required
1 Unattached young adult	Adolescent separation from family Increasing involvement with peers Courtship
2 Newly married couple	Formation of marital system Becoming adults in relation to parents/in-laws Bringing together two separate families of origin
3 Family with young children	Accepting new member into system Taking on parenting roles Extended family members become grandparents, aunts, uncles
4 Family with adolescents	Consideration of mid-life and career issues Young person moving in and out of family system Awareness of grandparents' increasing age and need for care
5 Launching children	Renegotiation of marital subsystem to become closer Development of adult relationship between parents and grown children Adjusting to becoming in-laws of children's spouses Loss of own parents (if not at earlier stage) Becoming grandparents
6 Family in retirement and later life	Change in the role of breadwinner Loss of siblings, friends Death of one partner, leaving other alone Life review and preparation for own death Middle generation involvement in caring for grand-parents

If we consider a young couple at, say, stage 3, we see that they face the tasks of adapting to a new family member and their new parenting roles. At the same time their parents could well be at stage 5. Having recently launched their children into new family systems, they are adapting to the grandparent role and renegotiating their marital relationship. Similar connections could be made between other stages of the cycle. It is for this reason that the family's development is described as an unbroken cycle, without a beginning or end.

The work that has been done on the family life-cycle (and summarised here) has mainly concentrated on a rather narrow definition of what is "normal". It may be that this pattern only relates to middle-class families in western society. For example, working-class old people are more likely than middle-class old people to look back at a life of frustrated ambitions and disappointments (Abrams, 1980). They may, therefore, have greater difficulty in coping with the tasks of the final stage in the cycle. There are now also, as previously mentioned, far more families in single parent households than in the past. There are, too, some households made up of homosexual couples, and others where children may be brought up in a commune, relating to several different adults. Such families are at the present time exceptions, but it is important to recognise that family patterns are constantly changing (as we saw in Chapter 2 when we discussed the findings of Young and Wilmott), and knowledge may become rapidly outdated. It is for these reasons that Haley cautions that we consider the developmental stages as guidelines rather than rigid rules.

An understanding of a family's life stage will enable the CPN to appreciate the tasks facing both the family as a whole and the individual members. This does not necessarily entail involving the whole family in an assessment since much can be learned by gathering information concerning other family members in an interview with the individual client. However, there may be times when the CPN finds herself inexorably drawn into attempting to handle "disturbed family relationships" (Sladden, 1979), and the greater understanding she has of family systems, the more able she will be to help disentangle the situation.

Life-events

Life-events – events likely to arouse strong negative or positive emotions, and that involve change in an activity, role, relationship or idea (Brown and Harris, 1978) – occur to everyone throughout life. In addition, an event in the life of one person almost always has repercussions for those close to that person. Life-events can be divided into two broad groupings, although there is a certain amount of overlap between the two.

First, life-events may be *developmental*, that is, transitional stages through which most members of a society will generally move. The timing of some of these stages is often determined by custom, while others may be determined by biology and physiological maturation. As a result they may often be anticipated by the person and those close to them. Such life-events include: puberty, leaving home in early adulthood, marriage, childbirth, retirement, and bereavement in old age. The second group of life-events are *accidental*, that is those that could not have been predicted, for example, major illness, miscarriage, redundancy, sudden and unexpected loss of a spouse by death or marital breakdown, or even, more positively, an unexpected win on the pools.

All such events may arouse strong emotions, either negative or, more often in the case of developmental events, positive. Life-events have been linked to both schizophrenic breakdown and the onset of depression, possibly through the mechanism of stress (Brown and Harris, 1978). However, it is now thought that it is not simply the change inherent in the event that is significant in causing stress, but the meaning of that event to those involved. Change may force us to alter our "assumptive world", that is, the set of rarely questioned assumptions that we hold about our own world, our work, personal relationships, health, home and the future. When this assumptive world is challenged and threatened by an event, then clearly the way an individual thinks and feels about himself is also challenged. In his autobiographical account of his own breakdown, Sutherland tells how he knew that his wife was having an affair for many years, but he did not become severely depressed until he discovered that the man was one of his friends (Sutherland, 1977). It seems that his discovery held a particularly significant meaning for him, and thus threatened his assumptive world causing him to become acutely depressed.

Brown and Harris have shown that serious life-events – those that have the most far-reaching effects on the way a person thinks about his or her world – are more likely to bring about depression. Most often these events feature disappointment and loss, and usually have long-term implications, for example, bereavement or marital breakdown.

Miss M, aged 59, was referred to the CPN team by her general practitioner to whom she had gone complaining of feelings of listlessness, difficulty in sleeping, tearfulness, and a loss of interest in life. When the CPN met her it emerged that she had retired six months earlier. At the time she had welcomed retirement, having worked hard in the garment business as a machinist all her life. Shortly before she left, the factory in which she worked had been taken over by a new manager whom she disliked, and this had added to her wish to retire. Despite looking forward to retirement, Miss M thought very little about it before it happened. Initially she enjoyed the unfamiliar leisure, had appreciated not having to get up so early, and had kept herself occupied with other interests. Gradually, however, she had more and more difficulty in getting up in the mornings, and became less interested in going out. She began to resent having little money to spend, and looked forward with gloom to what seemed to her an empty future.

As a single woman with few friends and no intimates, Miss M clearly gained much more from work than merely a pay-packet. It had provided her with social contacts, a structure to her day and week, and a source of self-esteem. With retirement she had lost not only her job but also these other benefits. She had suffered a loss that had long-term implications. If we consider Miss M's assumptive world, which she appeared to question rarely, we can see that it had indeed been threatened. She had thought of herself as someone who worked regularly and found almost all her social contact in the work setting. Quite suddenly she had lost all this and was forced to think about herself in a very different way.

We learn how to cope with events and threats to our selves through previous experiences. However, when an individual encounters an unexpected problem or an obstacle to a long-awaited life-goal that cannot be dealt with by normal problem-solving techniques, a crisis may arise. The person is likely, at first, to attempt to employ previously successful methods, which may not be appropriate in this situation. He or she will then become increasingly disorganised and distressed as the adopted strategy fails to overcome this new difficulty. There may then be a search for alternative methods of tackling the problem. The more unfamiliar it is, the more likely it is that, like Miss M, a person will have some difficulty in finding a solution quickly.

Like individuals, families will also as they develop encounter situations that they have not met before. Some families may feel a need to reinstate a possibly unhealthy family homeostasis, and their solution to the perceived threat may inhibit individual members' personal growth. In other cases they may initially resort to previously established methods of dealing with problems. For example, the parents of a young girl may forbid her to go out with an older man, having previously successfully managed to influence whom she sees. However, if they do not recognise that she has become more rebellious and would like more autonomy, they may find that their methods drive her further from them, and increase the likelihood of her seeing men they consider unsuitable. In another family, a middle-aged man may react to his wife's life-threatening illness with the same businesslike approach that he adopts when making decisions at work. He does not allow himself to face the emotional threat or allow his wife to share her feelings with him. In these two examples the people involved are using ways of coping that are not adapted to the particular situation in which they find themselves. Such coping mechanisms have been described as *maladaptive*. Coping mechanisms that allow a person to grow and to develop a new set of responses to potential crises are called *adaptive*.

It is immediately following a sudden serious event that it appears an individual or family is most open to change. Crisis intervention theory recognises this opportunity for change concentrated into a fairly short period of time and argues that by intervening very rapidly it may be possible to help the individual or family to develop ways of coping that are adaptive rather than maladaptive. By the time families in crisis come to the attention of the mental health services they may have already passed the most open phase. However where CPNs are attached to primary health care teams, and can respond to referrals very quickly when necessary, they may be able to intervene at the earlier stage and hence prevent deterioration of the individual's mental health or the family's stability.

CPN Action

Various factors affect the type of therapy or care provided by CPNs for their clients. The most important of these is, of course, the type of problems identified by the client, the family and the CPN. However, CPNs will also select different methods depending on their own interests, philosophies of mental health and illness, and the skills they possess. Many will adopt an eclectic approach to their nursing care. We think that whatever type of intervention is used, the family and social context of the person's life should be continually borne in mind.

Assessment

Crucial to the provision of good nursing care is a comprehensive assessment of the unique problems presented by a unique individual and/or the family, and their life situation. There is little benefit to be gained by the CPN adopting a prescription of the kinds of areas to be covered by a nursing assessment. Instead the CPN team could, through discussions, draw up its own guidelines which may be used to provide a framework. The information in Table 4.2 is drawn from guidelines devised by Bloomsbury CPN service.

Point II in Table 4.2 refers to the client's description of the main current problem. This moves away from the use of a medical diagnosis towards a definition of the problem from the client's point of view. Although there could be an almost infinite number of ways in which clients' problems could be described, one possible system, which can also be used for data collection, divides them into the following groups:

- mood-related problems
- abnormal experiences
- drugs or alcohol
- interpersonal relationships
- financial/housing/employment
- behavioural disturbance
- recent loss or separation
- anxiety
- no mental health problem

Clearly some of these are closely related to psychiatric diagnoses, but the difference is that the starting point is the client and family's understanding of the problem, rather than the professional staff's definition.

Within the assessment there will be greater emphasis on some areas than others, depending on the client's problem. For example, if a client has an alcohol problem, a greater part of the assessment will be taken up by exploring his drinking pattern and history. This may sometimes not be possible at the first contact, since the client's confidence and trust must be gained. In other instances, the CPN may wish to use certain measures, for example, rating scales for depression, anxiety or phobias, to assess the problem more accurately. Just as it is important that each

Table 4.2 GUIDELINES FOR ASSESSMENT

I Source of referral
   reason for and process of referral
   why now?
   client's attitude to referral

II Client's description of main problem, duration, etc.
   psychological, physical and social difficulties
   previous help received, when and from whom
   social situation –
      employment
      housing

III Previous problems, hospitalisation, treatment, etc.

IV Family history
   client's view of family
   family and agencies as a system

V Personal history
   childhood and adolescence
   cultural background
   schooling
   employment
   financial situation – source of income
   psychosexual development
   marriage/cohabitation
   children
   significant others

VI Usual personality
   traits, habits, interests
   self-esteem
   usual mood
   coping resources
   alcohol/drug use

VII Observations during interview
   appearance, behaviour
   mood
   speech
   thinking, beliefs, memory
   orientation, concentration
   insight
   rapport

VIII Information from other sources

IX Summary of current problems

X Action plan

client is seen as a unique individual, so the assessment process must be flexible enough to cope with different clients in different situations.

The final stage of the assessment guidelines is, in fact, not assessment, but the *action plan*. This is, as far as possible, based on the problem areas and goals agreed by the CPN and client, and encompasses a plan of care designed to tackle the problems and achieve the goals. By having agreed the problem areas and the ways in which they may be addressed, the CPN can evaluate the care provided by reviewing the extent to which the goals have been met. If rating scales have been used they would be repeated to measure the degree of change. A systematic approach to the evaluation of care plans and the progress made is an extremely important element. With such information the action plan may be amended accordingly and the care and treatment altered. An evaluation of care also gives CPNs an extremely valuable tool that can be used in determining with the client the most appropriate time for discharge. For example, the care plan could contain the objective of the client reaching and maintaining a certain level of functioning. Once this goal has been achieved, and if there are no further objectives to be reached, discharge may be considered, with any necessary arrangements for re-referral if appropriate. It can often be difficult for CPNs to discharge clients without such a system.

It is now common to talk of a "holistic" approach to nursing assessment and care, indicating the need for a person to be seen and treated as a whole, with no clear divide between mind and body, rather than as a set of discrete parts. The approach also suggests that the person's relationships with family and the outside world are important in reaching any understanding of him or her as a complete being. CPNs are clearly in a good position to be able to incorporate this perspective into their assessments, and the above guidelines demonstrate this approach. However, a word of warning may be appropriate here. Annie Altschul has pointed out that no one individual knew her completely, and she intended to keep it that way! (CPNA conference paper, 1985.) She would certainly resist any future CPN attempting a total assessment of her. We must be careful not to confuse our endeavours to treat clients as total human beings with a potentially intrusive wish to know everything about them. The purpose of assessment must always be to provide the best possible care.

Intervention

Having carried out a full assessment, the CPN may decide to offer one of a range of different types of therapy. This could be family meetings or therapy, behaviour therapy, counselling (intensive or supportive), practical advice, drug administration and/ or monitoring, or health education. Often a combination of these is needed. In some cases the CPN may think that no intervention is indicated, or that a referral elsewhere would be more appropriate.

CPNs often describe themselves as offering counselling to their clients. Although this term may be used more often to describe work with people with emotional crises, anxiety or depression, rather than those with psychotic disturbances, many of the principles underlying counselling are relevant to all areas of a CPN's work. It is not within the scope of this book to enter into a detailed discussion of different counselling techniques or other clinical skills, but rather to reflect some of the key elements that could be relevant to a wide range of different types of intervention, and to pick out what may be particularly important aspects to those receiving care.

A walk-in, self-referral counselling service in Oxford has been researched by one of its own staff, with much of the evaluation being based on the reports of the centre's clients (Oldfield, 1983). Oldfield found that making initial contact with the service was often very difficult for potential clients, but that, using concepts drawn from crisis theory, the early stages would be when the person was most open to change. Counsellors attempted to give clients an opportunity for security and attachment, with the eventual aim of increasing autonomy, self-esteem and confidence.

In the follow-up study clients were asked what aspects of their therapy they had found particularly helpful. Many mentioned the benefits of the counsellor being understanding, helpful, friendly, caring or supportive, but at the same time detached and calm. In addition there was a high degree of consistency in the importance of the counsellor showing warmth and concern, "a person there who's prepared to listen". Those characteristics of the counsellors that the clients felt were unhelpful included being impassive, remote, or appearing to disapprove or "play a role". Interestingly, some clients felt that there was too much concentration on their past, when their problems were in the present. Oldfield suggests that if an examination of the past was thought to be an essential element in counselling, this may need to be fully explained to the client involved.

Several clients liked the friendly atmosphere and some felt especially positive about the centre. One ex-client commented (Oldfield, 1983, p. 87):

normalisation of personal/emotional problems ... the idea of a chain of such "stress shops" into which people could walk and seek help with life-tasks they are confronted with, would be a major advance in moving from a system which focuses on mental illness, to one concerned with mental health.

We must not be too hasty in jumping to conclusions from this study, since it was based on fewer than half those who attended the centre during the research period (52 followed-up out of 144 attenders). Follow-up studies are likely to get a higher response rate from those who have fairly positive feelings about the service under review. In addition, this study excluded those who had attended fewer than four times, and we may speculate that such people could have been less satisfied with what they were offered than those who attended frequently.

Despite these reservations this study has important implications for CPNs. Many of its findings are reflected in other studies of the therapeutic relationship and, more importantly for CPNs, in a large-scale research project which compared the work of CPNs with that of psychiatrists in an out-patient department (Paykel and Griffith, 1983).

This study used various measures to compare, over 18 months, two randomly assigned groups of people with neuroses who required follow-up care after discharge from in-patient or day hospital care, or who were already being seen in the out-patient department. One group was seen by a psychiatrist in the out-patient department, while the other group was followed up by CPNs. One of the measures used was an assessment of the patient's satisfaction with the care received. Both groups felt fairly satisfied, but the researchers found that there was a general tendency for greater satisfaction among the CPN group. The nurses were more often described as easy to talk to, interested, kind, pleasant, making the patient feel relaxed, caring about the patient and better at their jobs than were the psychiatrists. The global satisfaction ratings also showed a difference between the two groups with satisfaction being greater within the CPN group. This difference was quite marked and reached a level of statistical significance when it was assessed at 12 and 18 months into the research. At 18 months none of the people being followed up by the CPNs would have preferred ordinary out-patient care, although many of them had had such care in the past. Many said that they liked being visited at home since the greater informality enabled them to develop a more confiding relationship with the nurse. However, a few felt that home visiting was intrusive and stigmatising in the eyes of family and neighbours.

Interestingly the nurses also appeared to convey more information to their clients than the psychiatrists did, but the researchers point out that in both groups the level of information was disappointingly low.

Many of the characteristics of the CPNs that were valued by their clients are similar to those described in the Oxford study as useful in a counselling relationship, for example warmth, concern and interest – aspects that are important in much of a CPN's work with a wide range of clients and problems. The suggestion is that if CPNs attempt to adopt many of the sometimes less flexible ways of working used by some psychiatrists, psychotherapists and others – for example, fixed appointment systems, waiting lists or a more remote demeanour – they may lose many of the elements of their therapeutic work most valued by their clients. In addition, it is now thought that counselling or psychotherapy is more likely to benefit someone if the therapist is from a similar cultural or class background. This again may prove to be a previously unrecognised strength of CPNs. Many clients, seeing nurses as coming from a relatively similar background to themselves, may find it easier to relate to them than they do to doctors.

Different Client Groups

We have made some general observations on the CPN's role in working with individuals and their families. We would now like to take this further. The work of CPN services is quite commonly discussed in terms of a division between short-term counselling or crisis work, and lengthier supportive work with those who may have long-standing problems. In fact this division is necessarily arbitrary, and the line between the two groups may become increasingly blurred in the future as more care is provided in community settings. However, for the sake of clarity, it is helpful to consider separately two broad groups who are often referred to CPNs: the long-term client group and the short-term or medium-term client group. This section will then also examine other groups with whom the CPN has an important role to play.

The long-term client group

Many CPN teams were first established to provide care for hospital patients discharged to live in the community who needed ongoing support or supervision. This is still a large part of the work of most teams. Many such clients have had schizophrenic or other psychotic illnesses, but in some cases their problems may now be as much to do with a lack of the skills needed to live in present-day society as it is to do with their original psychiatric condition. This is likely to be the case particularly with those who may be moving into community settings after many years of residence in large psychiatric hospitals. The move towards community care also means that in future fewer people will be admitted to hospital in the first place, or their stay there will be shorter than has been the case up to now. Dr Douglas Bennett has suggested that care in the community will not take away any of a person's underlying psychiatric disability, but will, if it is good care, remove the handicaps associated with institutional care, for example, stigma, poverty, isolation from the rest of society and lack of social skills. ("On the Move" Conference talk, 1985). He adds that those people with long-term needs will continue to require shelter, support and structure, although these will no longer be provided in one location. Both the relocation of long-stay hospital patients and the moves not to admit so readily in the future will have an impact on the work of nurses in the community.

The adoption of a nursing system that utilises the stages of assessment, planning, implementation and evaluation of care, such as we discussed earlier, could pose a potential problem for nurses working with this client group, since it implicitly identifies change and negotiation as the goals. What are the CPN's aims for someone who is perhaps severely damaged by a major psychiatric illness and for whom there is little prospect of change once he has reached a certain level of functioning? The answer lies in the concept of the tertiary level of prevention and the rehabilitative process (Table 4.3).

We shall discuss tertiary prevention first because, as CPN services develop and provide follow-up care from hospital, this is almost always the area in which they first operate. The area of secondary preventive work has been developed more recently and is discussed later in this chapter. The most recent – primary prevention – is discussed in Chapter 5.

Table 4.3   PREVENTION

Level of prevention	Aims	Model of care or treatment
Primary	Reducing the incidence of mental ill-health in the general population.	Health education/ promotion in groups; raising awareness.
Secondary	Reducing the duration of recognised mental ill-health; preventing long-term problems.	Early detection; effective, responsive, active treatment.
Tertiary	Preventing long-term handicap or disability as a result of mental illness.	Rehabilitation; maintenance of optimum level of functioning.

Tertiary prevention is the prevention of defect or handicap in people with a recognised condition (Caplan, 1969). At times this may mean an active rehabilitation programme which aims to markedly improve a person's social functioning, life skills and hence the quality of life. At other times, if someone has reached his optimum level of functioning, the goal may be maintenance of that improvement, rather than great change. In both these areas of work the CPN has a great deal to offer. The absence of clearly visible change in her clients should not lead the CPN or her manager to assume that her work is not extremely valuable.

Miss F was referred to the CPN by staff of the local day hospital where she had been attending erratically until recently but had now stopped attending altogether. A woman in her mid-30s, she lived on her own in a small, neglected flat. Miss F had gone to Oxford University after leaving school, gained a good degree, and got a job as a lecturer in a polytechnic teaching chemistry. After two years in this job she had a serious psychotic breakdown, was diagnosed as schizophrenic and lost her job. Now she lived an extremely isolated life, and spent much of her time ruminating on her ideas that she was being persecuted by members of the Mafia and the Conservative Party. She had become unable to follow her academic interests and had become estranged from her widowed mother who lived nearby.

After carrying out an assessment and discussing this with the day hospital team, the CPN decided that her main aim would be to help Miss F to be freer of some of her very distressing thoughts, and to be less socially isolated. This entailed attempting to establish a relationship of trust and to provide the right level of stimulation so that Miss F felt able to engage in activities rather than withdrawing completely as she had done in the past. After some time it was possible to reintroduce Miss F to the day hospital where she gradually developed an interest in art. Much later she followed this up herself by enrolling for an art class at the local adult education institute. With our current state of knowledge, Miss F is someone in whom we may not expect change very quickly, although over a period of time – perhaps years – the quality of her life may gradually improve. However, she is someone who indeed requires care aimed at the prevention of permanent disability, and this tertiary preventive care may be needed long-term.

In districts where there are CPNs particularly concerned with rehabilitation, their responsibilities would include follow-up after discharge, supervision of treatment including medication, support of the family (where they are involved), and prevention of relapse (Drake, 1981). In districts where there is an active policy of a transition to community care, the role of the CPN could be particularly central. (The 1985 CPNA Survey revealed that there were 42 CPNs working in this field.) CPNs could become actively involved in rehabilitation programmes prior to the client's discharge from hospital, concentrating especially on aspects of the transition which may cause difficulties or stress – anxieties about accommodation, transport and travelling, social security benefits, meeting the new neighbours and so on. The CPN would also assess the need for occupation and daytime structured activities. If the client is moving into unstaffed accommodation the CPN could then continue the support established within the hospital once the person is discharged.

In Italy, where a number of mental health policies have been pioneered, nurses working in the community are often involved in intensive programmes of rehabilitation with a much smaller number of clients than CPNs would be in Britain. Such practices may mean that they sometimes have to work more flexible hours in order to be able to visit clients at times when they may need the most help, for example, early in the morning or over a weekend (Brooker, 1985b).

In addition to practical support, counselling may also be extremely beneficial to such clients. A person who has suffered a major psychiatric illness may need a great deal of support in learning to cope with the consequences. Just as someone who has diabetes will with help learn to live with the problem, so may someone with, for example, schizophrenia. They may come to recognise triggers or situations which aggravate their problems, and their way of dealing with these may be selective withdrawal to prevent becoming over-stimulated (Ekdawi, 1981). The problems that beset those with long-standing conditions are, of course, both protracted and also prone to become more marked with life-events and setbacks, to which they are more vulnerable than others. For this reason Ekdawi recommends two main elements to rehabilitation counselling:

- Continuity and stability to help the client to tackle the long-term difficulties.
- Availability and flexibility at times of emergency.

Topics raised in sessions might include:

- The client's need for clear information.
- His thoughts about his future.
- How to deal with abnormal experiences.
- The need for medication.
- Side-effects.
- What to tell potential employers.
- Interpersonal problems.
- Problems with social security benefits.

Although many of the general principles of counselling will be relevant to rehabilitation counselling, CPNs in this field will also need considerable knowledge of the psychiatric conditions that can cause long-term problems.

Some CPN teams, particularly those covering inner-city areas, may find that many people referred to their service have little or no contact with their families and little other support. When 100 patients in a large London mental hospital were interviewed, it was found that half of them expected to sleep, sit or do nothing for most of the day once they were discharged, 80% felt lonely, nearly 50% said they had no one to turn to for advice or support, and most had no friends (McCowan and Wilder, 1976). As we saw in Chapter 2 the rates of schizophrenia are higher in inner-city areas, as it is thought that people may leave the place where they grew up and drift into the cities perhaps for somewhere to live or work or to find anonymity. Other clients may have lost contact with family and friends through their prolonged or repeated admissions to hospital. Many of those who have, or have had, psychiatric illnesses have smaller social networks and less opportunity for personal intimacy than others. People who are rootless and perhaps homeless provide a particular challenge to CPNs, and the nurse's work will often bring her into contact with voluntary agencies working with this group.

In a review of the clients referred to her from a hostel for homeless women, Wadsworth (1984) found that they fell into three groups. One group had clear signs of psychiatric disturbance, but refused any offer of help or assessment. A second group had often had a long history of contact with psychiatric services and may have been seen by a CPN before. They would be willing to see the CPN and possibly also a psychiatrist and would often take medication for a short time. However, they would usually not stay very long in the hostel and would not maintain contact when they moved on. It is especially important that accurate records are kept on such people, since, as Wadsworth points out, they frequently return to the same hostel or one in the same area months or even years later. The third group tended to be younger women often with backgrounds of emotional deprivation and separations; some would have a history of short admissions to psychiatric hospital perhaps for self-harm. The CPN's role with such diverse clients must necessarily be varied, but in all cases it entails close liaison and cooperation with the hostel or voluntary agency staff. In many cases the CPN's work will also involve supporting hostel staff in what is often a stressful job and, of course, acting as an information resource for them.

At the beginning of this chapter we discussed how the meeting of many different needs (including belonging to a group, support and recognition) contributes to a person's mental health. However, we also saw that, without certain basic requirements – shelter, food, warmth – being met, it is much more difficult for the individuals or the CPN to address issues more obviously related to mental health.

Many CPNs who work with homeless people have discovered that while someone lives on the streets it is almost impossible to engage him in, say, counselling, without also addressing the issues of his homelessness and lack of money. It will sometimes be more appropriate for the CPN who knows him to help him to sort out his financial situation and find somewhere to live, than to involve another professional who more usually deals with such matters.

In some districts the provision of long-term accommodation outside the hospital that can provide some support to residents who have had major psychiatric illness has become a health authority responsibility. In one such scheme a CPN was responsible for a small number of group homes (Leopoldt, 1980). She would visit each home weekly, often in the evening in order to see all the residents. Her work would include monitoring and administering medication, assessing and supporting individual residents, and helping residents to explore and resolve any group tensions. She would also liaise with general practitioners, psychiatrists, social workers and employers.

Clearly such work, focused as it is around housing, requires a good working relationship between the CPN and other agencies, including advice centres, social security offices, social services and so on. However, this is also the case wherever CPNs look beyond the narrow confines of psychiatric illness and symptomatology to encompass wider aspects of mental health. We shall return to the subject of liaison with other workers in Chapter 6.

In this discussion of the care of long-term clients we have not yet mentioned medication. Medication, particularly the neuroleptics or major tranquillisers, is an important element in the treatment of many with psychiatric disorders. These drugs can have a marked antipsychotic and, in some cases, a sedative effect. They have enabled many people to live normal lives outside of a hospital setting and made it possible for others to have a better quality of life less disturbed by their psychotic experiences. Depôt medication gives the clients who receive it an even drug–blood level. It is also often preferred for those who may forget to take oral medication regularly, since it can be easily monitored.

Despite these advantages there is, however, increasing disquiet among some professionals, some recipients of such medication and members of the public about its side-effects. As we know, phenothiazines can cause parkinsonian-like symptoms, weight gain, atropine-like effects and tardive dyskinesia. The latter may not disappear once the drug is stopped and may even become more marked and disabling if the major tranquilliser is reduced. Nevertheless, for many people a drug regime can be devised that does not cause discomfort. Many of these people will be living in their own homes and possibly being given depôt medication by a CPN.

We hope that our discussions so far have shown that the CPN's role may be much more far-reaching than the straightforward administration of medication. However, we also suggest that the CPN is one of the best-placed professionals to take on a monitoring and reviewing role, in conjunction with the prescribing medical officer, of the levels and side-effects of medication that may be both extremely therapeutic, but also potentially quite damaging.

Short-term and medium-term CPN work

At the beginning of their research into the work of CPNs, Paykel and Griffith (1983) made the point that CPNs were not accustomed to taking on clients who had neurotic rather than psychotic disorders. In their area such people had more commonly been seen by psychiatrists or possibly by their GPs. There may still be districts where this continues to be the case, but in many areas CPNs are now taking referrals of people with a wide range of different problems.

A large part of this development has come about through CPNs working more closely with primary health care workers and encouraging referrals direct from GPs and other community nurses. Much of the CPN's work will still involve rehabilitation, follow-up support and perhaps the administration of medication for people who have recognised psychiatric illnesses, but a link with a primary health care team allows the CPN to also practise secondary prevention (see Table 4.3).

Secondary prevention refers to early detection enabling early intervention and the prevention of further deterioration or of the client developing a recognised psychiatric illness (Caplan, 1969). This is facilitated by CPN services having greater community links since people with problems may be picked up much more quickly at the first indications of anything being wrong. They may also be much more willing to see someone who works from their local health centre than they would be to attend the psychiatric hospital, since there is no inherent stigma with the former. One small psychiatric team (including a CPN) was attached to a health centre (Corser and Ryce, 1977). Their report mentions a 97% attendance rate for psychiatric appointments, and claims that this high level is because of the accessibility and lack of stigma. Interestingly the same study found that health visitors and district nurses who were based in the same health centre became more confident in dealing with mental health problems themselves as a result of their contact with the CPN.

Clients who are referred by primary health care workers may have had no previous contact with psychiatric services, and may require quite different types of CPN intervention from those with major psychiatric illness. In some instances they and their families may be experiencing a life crisis or emotional trauma and need some brief but intensive help to find their own solutions. With this group the nurse working in the community is likely to employ more intensive counselling or family therapy.

Mr T was referred to the CPN by his general practitioner, with whom the CPN worked closely. He had attended the surgery complaining of sleeplessness, an inability to continue his job as a storeman because of exhaustion and depression, an increased frequency of arguments with his wife, and being at the "end of his tether" with his mother. He and his wife were seen together by the nurse and a detailed assessment carried out. They had been married for 20 years, were very close and had no children. His mother lived in a council flat nearby and was crippled by severe arthritis so that she needed almost constant nursing care. This care was provided almost entirely by Mr T and his wife dividing the day between them, since Mr T felt that it would be an abdication of responsibility for him to involve others. Recently his mother had become more disabled and more demanding. Shortly before this he had told her that he would like to go away for a weekend and she had been very upset by the news. Her deteriorating health and his feelings of guilt had precipitated his depression and inability to cope.

The nurse offered Mr T appointments for counselling in which he was able to explore his feelings about his sometimes domineering mother, his relationship with his wife and their childlessness, and his need to see himself as providing all the care to his mother. After four sessions he was able to plan the weekend away that he had talked of before, and felt happy to leave his mother's care in the hands of a cousin. He and his wife began to go out together occasionally, something they had hardly done for five years. He also gradually introduced to his mother the idea of a brief admission to hospital so that he and his wife could have a fortnight's holiday. To his evident relief, after approximately five weeks, Mr T reported an improvement in his relationship with his wife and, to his surprise, with his mother.

Over the course of this Mr T had three weeks off sick from his job. He required no medication and felt fully restored to his normal self by the time he was discharged. A potential family crisis, that could have resulted among other things in the inappropriate admission of Mr T's mother to hospital had been averted.

With other clients, the CPN may find it appropriate to offer behaviour therapy. (A number of those trained as nurse behaviour therapists work as members of CPN teams, but it is of course also a therapy used by others. For a discussion on the differences between nurse therapists and CPNs see Brooker (1985a); also Barker (1982) and Marks *et al.* (1977).)

> Mrs R had had no previous contact with psychiatric services when she went to her doctor complaining of her increasing difficulty in going out alone. When the CPN met her, he discovered that Mrs R had become more and more isolated since her divorce 18 months earlier. Around that time she had started to experience anxiety when going out into open spaces, using lifts or crossing busy roads, and had gradually limited her movements in order to cope. By the time she was seen by the CPN she was suffering great anxiety and described having had panic attacks when confronted with the need to make a journey beyond her immediate neighbourhood. Together the CPN and Mrs R agreed on a programme of behaviour therapy, with a series of graded tasks which Mrs R would do with the nurse, a close friend or on her own. The CPN taught Mrs R some relaxation techniques that could be used in any situation. Over the course of several weeks Mrs R was able to tackle most of the agreed tasks, but was still unable to use lifts in public buildings. She felt that this was not a major problem and did not wish to continue with the programme further. Several months later she suffered a temporary setback when a close friend moved away and, in anticipation of a recurrence of her previous problems, she contacted the CPN. After only two sessions Mrs R felt able to cope once again, but appreciated being able to contact the nurse in the future if she wished.

As well as facilitating the early detection of mental health problems, links with primary health care workers can also enable the CPN to carry out other work. For the GP or health visitor the CPN can be an invaluable link with the hospital psychiatric services, often acting in a recognised liaison role, but also at times opening up channels of communication for others to use. As a result of their knowledge of admission systems and their flexible patterns of working, CPNs can play an active part in paving the way for hospital admission if in their opinion someone referred to them requires it. This may result in a client being admitted to hospital with less delay, and with the ward staff having more information about the client than is usual.

When CPN services widen the range of people or agencies who may refer to them they will almost certainly find that some of those referred do not require the resources of a CPN, but need something provided elsewhere. CPNs based in community settings require a good knowledge of other services in the area and should be willing to refer a new client to another agency if that is more appropriate. (We shall return to the subject of a CPN's work with other professionals in Chapter 6.) Similarly, closer links with other community workers often lead to the nurse acting as a consultant to colleagues. The CPN may be asked by a district nurse to accompany her on a visit to someone who is causing her anxiety. As someone who may have known the family concerned for several years, the district nurse may not wish to refer to the CPN formally but would appreciate some advice on a new family development. The CPN's role may well be two-fold: to give clinical advice on the best way for the district nurse to provide nursing care and to provide peer support in what may be a highly stressful situation. In other cases advice and information may be provided without the CPN seeing the client, perhaps through a regular liaison meeting or through informal contact. As we mentioned earlier, health visitors and district nurses in a health centre felt more confident to deal with mental health problems once they had access to a CPN. This is a model that could be developed in many areas.

The brief of mental health services as a whole has been widened over the past few decades, so that problems that were previously conceptualised as "life problems" have become potential reasons for psychiatric treatment. The term "worried well" has been coined to describe those people who might now ask for counselling, whereas before they may have turned to friends and family. There has been concern that people may have excessive expectations of counselling, and that they may wish to use it to absolve themselves of responsibility for their own lives. However, various community studies have highlighted significant levels of mental distress in the general population (see, for example, Brown and Harris, 1978), and these could be precursors of more serious problems later on. It is our belief that CPNs working in community settings, in a way that is accessible to a larger section of society, may be able to contribute to the early detection and alleviation of such distress, and hence the prevention of the consequences.

Clients with drug or alcohol problems

Although some districts may now have specialist drug or alcohol services (some with CPNs), it is arguably the responsibility of all the caring professionals to offer some help to those with drug or alcohol problems.

There has been a huge increase in both drug and alcohol use in recent years, with an explosion in heroin use in particular. The increase in alcohol problems has been less visible, probably because of the social acceptability of drinking. However, it is thought that between 20% and 25% of all those in general hospital medical beds have an illness caused by alcohol consumption, although this is often not detected (Davies and Raistrick, 1981). The greatest increase in problem drinking has been among women, possibly because of increased availability, relatively cheaper price and, again, increased acceptability.

For CPNs not working in specialist services their greatest contribution will be in early detection, health education and in offering a range of therapy, family meetings and support to those concerned about their heavy drinking. This would be done in close collaboration with the client's general practitioner and any other professionals involved. A good knowledge of local specialist agencies, in both the statutory and voluntary sectors, will enable the nurse to refer to specialists when appropriate.

Old people

We have not until now specifically referred to the CPN's work with elderly people. This has been quite deliberate, since many of the problems that old people face are very similar to those of younger people, and hence much of what has been written will be relevant to them. However, it is important to recognise that work with the elderly is the most common CPN speciality (currently one CPN in five; CPNA, 1985), and for those who carry a generic caseload old people will make up a significant proportion of it.

We saw in Chapter 2 that many old people live alone, and are often very isolated. Only 6% of elderly people live in any form of residential care with the rest living in their own homes. Many old people will have seen huge changes in society, social attitudes and values, as well as in the environment, during the course of their lives. Some old people will "disengage" from society and will avoid new experiences in order to cope with these changes. Old age is not a problem in itself, but is a life-stage which requires quite major adjustments to changes in health and vigour, income, family roles, employment, and friendships. Old people may suffer from the same mental health problems as younger people, but in addition they are more prone to develop confusional states, often related to physical illness or medication; paranoid states (possibly related to social isolation or deafness); and senile dementia. The CPN, alongside other professionals, has a very important part to play in the mental health care of old people.

Mr K was admitted to the psychiatric ward of the district general hospital having been found wandering the streets at night wearing only his dressing-gown. He said that he was looking for his wife, although she had died six weeks earlier. He was severely disoriented, and appeared to have been neglecting himself. The ward staff asked the CPN to become involved almost immediately, since the subsequent diagnoses of senile dementia and malnutrition indicated that, should Mr K return home, he would almost certainly need continuing care. The general practitioner pointed out that prior to her sudden death Mrs K had carried out almost all of the household tasks, and nursed her husband devotedly. It was discovered that the flat was extremely dirty, with decomposing food in it. Mr K had not been collecting his pension, and had no money at all.

It was felt by several members of the multidisciplinary team that staffed residential accommodation would be the most appropriate for Mr K, but he adamantly refused to consider leaving his flat. Finally, a professional network was established consisting of the social worker, CPN, meals-on-wheels coordinator, home help, and day centre staff, with the CPN taking on the role of key worker. A series of gradually lengthening visits home were arranged, with a member of staff accompanying Mr K each time. After several weeks, he was discharged home. On almost every day he would be seen by at least one member of the network, and regular meetings of those involved (convened by the CPN) ensured that any deterioration or other change in his condition would be quickly picked up. The staff involved were keenly aware that there was a risk in Mr K living alone at home, but felt that this was justified in the light of his clearly expressed wish to stay.

In Chapter 1 we discussed how community mental health services and CPN services should be underpinned by a number of principles including the following: an individual's right to be cared for at home whenever possible, care which should aim to decrease dependence and maintain the right to make choices; and care which should be based on individual needs. In the case of Mr K it would perhaps have been easier, and safer, to have strongly encouraged him to move into residential accommodation or even to have kept him in hospital. However, it appears that the action taken, after careful consideration and planning, was instead guided by such principles.

The family's role in caring

What about those people with long-term or short-term problems who have families with whom they may either be living, or having regular contact? Two separate but related themes are particularly relevant to the CPN caring for such clients and their families: (a) the role of the family in caring for the ill member, and the consequent burden they experience; (b) the part played by family atmosphere, levels of emotion, and intensity of contact in influencing the relapse rate for people with diagnoses of schizophrenia, and the application of research on these factors to the work of CPNs.

Family burden

Many writers in considering the moves towards community care have acknowledged the importance of the family (see, for example, Walker, 1982). In caring for people discharged after a long admission, families may carry much of the burden of care; and Wing (1981) argues that they should be helped by the provision of crisis help, holiday relief, and a range of occupational, leisure and residential facilities. Without such help it is conceivable that some families may come to question the desirability of community care, as they see services being provided primarily to those who do not have families, and they may feel themselves penalised for caring (Moroney, 1976).

What, then, is meant by "family burden"? Several different effects have been described, including disturbances to relatives' health, to social and leisure activities and domestic routine, effects on children in the household, and reduction in income (Grad and Sainsbury, 1963). It has been suggested that families of those referred to CPN services may well experience such stresses, and may not previously have had access to support (Sladden, 1979). However, in their evaluative study of the work of CPNs with people with neurotic disorders, Paykel and Griffith (1983) found that, for the small proportion of the two comparison groups who had a close relative, such relatives tended to report very low levels of family burden. The researchers suggested that this may be due to the fact that the clients very seldom, if ever, behaved abnormally at home. Clearly, family burden is likely to be higher when a family member has had a psychotic episode and may be behaving in a disturbed way. Some research in this area has reported that family members' "subjective" reports of their burden are considerably lower than the researchers' "objective" ratings from questionnaires (see, for example, Hoenig and Hamilton, 1966). Similarly, people who live with, or feel responsible for, someone with a diagnosis of schizophrenia, may understate their problems despite there being major effects on their lives (Creer and Wing, 1974). In this study family carers complained that their ill relatives were underactive, uncommunicative, slow and had no leisure interests. The writers suggest that the carers had nevertheless become accustomed to their situations, and had accordingly adjusted their own hopes and aspirations downwards.

In contrast to the studies that report lower levels of family burden than one might have expected, we have found that, using research methods that attempt to get closer to the carers' understanding of their situation, relatives are indeed aware of how different their lives are from those of others, and of the responsibilities they shoulder (Simmons, 1984).

Several of the interviewees in this research were considerably affected by their psychologically disturbed relative. Some had become isolated, and felt unable to mix socially or go away for a holiday. Some felt the strain in terms of a deterioration in their own physical or mental health, and most had contributed financially to their relative's income. In the case of close relatives (for example, spouse, parent or child), this appears to be accepted as part of the relationship. However, where the relationship has not contained elements of mutual support or reciprocal interchange in the past, for example, in the case of siblings or in-laws, family members were more likely to see it purely as a burdensome duty, and feel consequently resentful. Particularly when she feels she receives nothing back, the carer may withdraw from the situation to protect her own psychological wellbeing (Gottlieb, 1983).

What then are the implications of these studies for CPNs? One conclusion is that it is important that we pay more attention to what family members tell us about their situation. Many are not used to being asked about their own experiences, only about the person who has been identified as having the problem. We do not recognise sufficiently often that relatives are acting as the primary family carers, with health and social services as back-ups. CPNs could therefore play a very important role in providing support. This may be particularly beneficial where there is little involvement from other members of the family, since we know that those who experience high levels of stress, such as in the day-to-day care of a psychiatrically ill relative, are less likely to develop poor health themselves if they have access to a significant other or social intimate (Gottlieb, 1983). Although a CPN cannot become a social intimate in the sense meant by Gottlieb, her emotional and interpersonal support of a family carer may counteract the imbalance in the family system whereby the carer gets little back from the person receiving the care. Indeed, Gottlieb suggests that it may be more feasible to increase the support to primary carers, rather than to decrease significantly the stressors that they experience.

High expressed emotion (HEE)

As well as looking at family members' experiences of caring, it has also been fruitful to examine the possible influences of the family on the course of psychiatric conditions. This can be thought of as an interaction between certain family processes and the course of established psychiatric illnesses. If these processes can be identified it may be possible to influence their course, reduce their detrimental effect, and hence improve the quality of life of both the client and family. The work in this area has focused on the levels of expressed emotion within family interaction and has particularly highlighted two elements of this: criticism and over-involvement (Brown, Birley and Wing, 1972; Vaughn and Leff, 1976). People who have had a schizophrenic breakdown and return to live in a family where they receive a high level of criticism and/or one or more members of their family are over-involved with them, have been found to be more likely to relapse than those in low expressed emotion households. The effects of high expressed emotion (HEE) appear to be modified by a reduction in the actual hours of face-to-face contact, and by medication. Low expressed emotion does not simply refer to an absence of involvement, but to a positive, but non-intrusive concern.

There are clear implications of these studies for the work of CPNs. We do not have to know the causes of schizophrenia to be able to influence its course by applying some of these findings.

Some work has attempted to reduce the level of expressed emotion in HEE families by: a combination of education of family carers on the nature of schizophrenia; what to expect and how to respond; the provision of emergency access by telephone; involving the family in the planning of the client's care; and setting up relatives' groups within which high and low expressed emotion carers were mixed. In these groups it has been found that relatives are more able to take advice and criticism from each other than from professionals (Priestley, 1979). Hence those who would normally be very critical of the person they are caring for may learn different ways of approaching situations from other people who have experienced similar problems.

When such groups are not appropriate or possible, a few key strategies may be helpful to family carers. Kuipers (quoted in Shepherd, 1984) suggests the following guidelines:

- set clear rules and standards
- coax sympathetically, do not pressurise
- know when to ignore behaviour
- do not argue with delusions, accept subjective reality, while not agreeing with objective truth
- use distractions
- use humour occasionally

Where it is not possible to reduce the level of criticism or involvement, it may then be preferable to attempt to alter the hours of contact. Of course this is sometimes done anyway by the client adopting a different lifestyle from the rest of the family, perhaps sleeping during the day and staying up all night, or locking himself away in his room for periods of the day. Such methods may provide some relief, but also prevent the person receiving the level of stimulation and social contact that he needs. A much better alternative would be some activity that took the client out of the house during the day. In some cases this may be provided by work, but for many it means attendance at a day centre, day hospital, or workshop. It seems that most particularly at risk are young, unmarried men living with parents who demonstrate a high level of expressed emotion (Vaughn and Leff, 1976), and may particularly need the protection of reduced contact and medication. For CPNs and others involved in their care this may require a great deal of continuing work to encourage a client who may at times be very reluctant to carry on attending.

The following is a final illustration of the family's caring role:

David W was referred to his local CPN by the psychiatric out-patient department. He was 48 years old, and lived with his mother and father who were 72 and 78 respectively. The family had only recently moved into the area having been rehoused by the council in a ground-floor flat because of Mrs W's decreasing mobility. Following an acute psychotic breakdown in his teens, David W spent 18 years in a large psychiatric hospital. Originally it had been thought that he would never leave the hospital, but the medical staff had eventually suggested it when he responded well to medication. His parents were delighted to have him home, and ever since his father had devoted his life to looking after him. This involved cooking his meals, doing all the housework, buying his clothes and cigarettes, and liaising with hospital staff and the family's general practitioner. Since having a stroke five years ago Mrs W had also needed more nursing care, including a great deal of lifting, and Mr W divided his time between the two.

The original referral was made to the CPN for her to give David his three-weekly depôt medication. However, in the course of her assessment the CPN found that there were several other issues to be addressed. Mr W (senior) was feeling particularly overstretched by the increasing demands on him. He had not had any time off for several months, and had not had a holiday for years. His great love was bowling and he used to go regularly with an old friend. Both parents were becoming concerned about who would care for their son as their own health deteriorated and when they would eventually die. Although the family atmosphere was rarely highly charged or critical, there was certainly a degree of over-involvement between the parents and their son.

Over the course of several months the CPN was able to establish a relationship of trust between herself and the three members of the family. David was encouraged to attend a local day centre. Initially he would only go if he was accompanied by his father or, on a few occasions, by the CPN, but later he attended on his own, and through the centre renewed his former interest in woodwork. Once David was well-established there his parents were prepared to consider a short holiday for themselves, and this was arranged through a voluntary organisation for elderly people. In addition, Mr W spent several half-days bowling with his friend. As well as considering David's occupational need, and the needs of his parents, the CPN was also aware that it would be important to consider possible future housing for David. Gradually she was able to introduce the idea of a supportive hostel or group-home to David and his parents. Although none of them was prepared to consider a move at this stage, the fact that the idea had been introduced would make it easier for it to be reconsidered if, in the future, the parents' failing health necessitated it.

The CPN's nursing care plan had acknowledged the importance of the family in caring for their son, and had also gone further in attempting to address the family members' needs in addition to David's. There was a recognition too that although David and his parents would require CPN help for perhaps years to come, this did not mean that change was not possible or not worth striving for. Such change would necessarily be gradual but could significantly increase the quality of all their lives.

Summary

In this chapter we have briefly examined what is meant by mental health, introduced the concept of the family as a system, and looked at the relevance of life-events and transitions in people's lives to the work of CPNs. We then went on to discuss various aspects of the CPN's work including the importance of assessment, and nursing care planning. In the section on particular client groups we have emphasised working with individuals and their families, including those with long-term needs and those who require short-term intervention. We have also discussed the family's role in caring as this becomes an increasingly important element in community care. Throughout the chapter we have put forward a case for CPNs working with a psychosocial model in which they take into account the immediate environment of the client's life, as well as the problem that he or she presents. In the next chapter we shall broaden our perspective to encompass, in addition, the wider society.

References

Abrams, M. (1980) *Beyond Three-score and Ten. 2nd report.* Age Concern Publications, Mitcham.

Anderson, M. (1971) *Sociology of the Family.* Penguin, Harmondsworth.

Barker, P. J. (1982) *Behaviour Therapy Nursing.* Croom Helm, London.

Brooker, C. (1985a) Two psychiatric entities. *Nursing Mirror,* **9 January,** 35–6.

Brooker, C. (1985b) Community mental health services in Italy. *Community Psychiatric Nursing Journal,* **5(3),** 11–18.

Brown, G. W., Birley, J. L. T. and Wing, J. K. (1972). The influence of family life on the course of schizophrenic disorders: a replication. *British Journal of Psychiatry*, **121**, 241–58.

Brown, G. W. and Harris, T. O. (1978) *The Social Origins of Depression*. Tavistock, London.

Carter, E. A. and McGoldrick, M. (1980) (eds) *The Family Life-Cycle: Framework for Family Therapy*. Gardner Press,

Caplan, G. (1969) *An Approach to Community Mental Health*. Tavistock, London.

Clare, A. (1976) *Psychiatry in Dissent*. Tavistock, London.

Corser, C. M. and Ryce, S. W. (1977) Community mental health care: a model based on the primary care team. *British Medical Journal*, **2**, 936–8.

Community Psychiatric Nurses Association (1985) *The 1985 CPNA National Survey Update*. CPNA Publications, Leeds.

Creer, C. and Wing, J. (1974) *Schizophrenics at Home*. National Schizophrenia Fellowship, Surbiton.

Davies, I. and Raistrick, D. (1981) *Dealing with Drink*. BBC Publications, London.

Drake, W. (1981) The role of the nurse: the community psychiatric nurse, in Wing, J. W. and Morris, B. (eds) *Handbook of Psychiatric Rehabilitation Practice*. Oxford University Press, Oxford.

Ekdawi, M. Y. (1981) Counselling in rehabilitation, in Wing, J. W. and Morris, B. (eds) *Handbook of Psychiatric Rehabilitation Practice*, Oxford University Press, Oxford.

Gottlieb, B. H. (1983) *Social Support Strategies*. Sage Publications, London.

Grad, J. and Sainsbury, P. (1963) Mental illness and the family. *Lancet*, **9 March,** 544–7.

Haley, J. (1973) *Uncommon Therapy: The Psychiatric Techniques of Milton H. Erikson*. Norton, New York.

Hoenig, J. and Hamilton, M. (1966) The schizophrenic patient in the community and his effect on the household. *International Journal of Social Psychiatry*, **12(3)**, 165–76.

Leopoldt, H. (1980) The psychiatric group home – 2. *Nursing Times*, **15 May,** 866–8.

McCowan, P. and Wilder, J. (1976) *The Lifestyle of One Hundred Psychiatric Patients*. Psychiatric Rehabilitation Association, London.

Marks, I. M., Halleron, R. S., Connolly, J. and Philpott, R. (1977) *Nursing in Behavioural Psychotherapy*. Royal College of Nursing, London.

Maslow, A. H. (1968) *Toward a Psychology of Being*. Van Nostrand Reinhold, New York.

Minuchin, S. (1974) *Families and Family Therapy*. Tavistock, London.

Moroney, R. M. (1976) *The Family and the State*. Longman, London.

Oldfield, S. (1983) *The Counselling Relationship*. Routledge and Kegan Paul, London.

Paykel, E. S. and Griffith, J. H. (1983) *Community Psychiatric Nursing for Neurotic Patients*. Royal College of Nursing, London.

Priestley, D. (1979) Schizophrenia and the family, in Wing, J. K. and Olsen, R. *Community Care for the Mentally Disabled*. Oxford University Press, Oxford.

Robinson, D. (1971) *The Process of Becoming Ill*. Routledge and Kegan Paul, London.

Shepherd, G. (1984) *Institutional Care and Rehabilitation*. Longman, Harlow.

Simmons, S. M. (1984) *Family burden – What does it mean to the carers?* Unpublished MSc dissertation, University of Surrey.

Sladden, S. (1979) *Psychiatric Nursing in the Community.* Churchill Livingstone, Edinburgh.

Sutherland, S. (1977) *Breakdown.* Paladin, London.

Vaughn, C. E. and Leff, J. P. (1976) The influence of family and social factors on the course of psychiatric illness. *British Journal of Psychiatry,* **129,** 125–37.

Wadsworth, R. (1984) Turning Point for the Homeless. *Nursing Times,* **80(44),** 48–9.

Walker, A. (ed.) (1982) *Community Care.* Blackwell and Robertson, Oxford.

Walrond-Skinner, S. (1977) *Family Therapy.* Routledge and Kegan Paul, London

Wing, J. W. (1981) From institutional to community care. *Psychiatric Quarterly,* **53(2),** 139–51.

5

The Role of the CPN with Groups and the Wider Society

Many CPNs are now incorporating a family perspective into their work with clients. In this chapter we shall look beyond the individual and the immediate family system, and consider the wider system of the local community and society. Humans are basically social beings living in a complex society, and the implications of this for mental health and the work of the CPN are manifold, as we shall see.

Defining Primary and Secondary Groups

In Chapter 4 we discussed how the family is generally the most important primary group of which the individual is a member. By *primary* group we mean those groups characterised by a high degree of face-to-face contact, and in many instances intimacy, or at least cooperation between the members. A person will generally be a member of several other primary groups in addition to his family, including school groups, friendship groups, occupational groups, societies, clubs, and church groups. Some of these will in turn form part of larger organisations – for example, trade unions, business companies, or colleges. Such larger organisational groups are sometimes referred to as *secondary* groups. Primary groups tend to be our chief source of social satisfaction. We learn what kind of person we are by observing, in group settings, the responses of others to us. Some primary groups may also be useful to society as a whole, or to a larger organisation of which they may be a part, through exercising some social control and encouraging a degree of conformity. In some cases, of course, this group conformity may work against the interests of the larger group, as, for example, where a small closely-knit group of young people may vandalise their own neighbourhood.

We also saw in Chapter 4 that Maslow's hierarchy of needs (see Fig. 4.1) identifies belongingness and love needs as ones that should be met in order for someone to be motivated by the higher level needs of self-esteem and the esteem of others, and to reach self-actualisation. For adults in particular the need to love, feel loved and liked, and to belong, will be met within other social groups in addition to their immediate family circle. So people will often seek out others who share similar ideas, life-styles or interests, and join up in formal or informal groups. Friendship groups provide acceptance, a sense of identity, affection, support and credibility to their members.

In earlier, less complex and less urbanised societies, primary groups would constitute most if not all of an individual's network. Those people with whom a man worked would also be the ones with whom as a child he went to school, and who would now be his neighbours. A woman would shop in the village grocery store run by people whose children she occasionally looked after, and with whom she also went to church. However, it has been suggested that the growing complexity of western urban society has led to a relative reduction in such primary group contacts, with a parallel increase in secondary groups (Pons, 1977). For some clients face-to-face contact with their CPN could well be a substitute for the lack of primary group interaction in their lives. Within a secondary group – for example, in a work environment – roles tend to be more clearly defined and rule-bound, and the group members come together for specific and limited purposes. This growth of secondary group activities is caused in part by a clear split between work and home life, both in terms of time allocation and geographical location, and in some areas housing redevelopment which has broken up old communities.

Integration and Disintegration

There has been in recent years growing concern about the impact of such changes on the mental health of communities. In writing about the industrial town of Salford, for example, one psychiatrist points out that prior to the major housing redevelopments of the 1960s and 1970s social groups tended to focus on familiar

streets, shops and other informal meeting places (Freeman, 1984).
Similarly, another writer examining life in small neighbourhoods
points out that "When there is considerable interaction between
neighbours the street, the court, the alley or the lane is more than
a mere aggregate of dwellings. The physical neighbourhood is
distinguished by its inhabitants as an entity" (Sprott, 1958). In
Salford at least, many of these neighbourhoods have been lost and
replaced by ugly tower blocks in which many people lead isolated
lives. In Chapter 2 we considered various factors which appear to
be related to mental health problems, including unemployment,
social class, housing and so on. Based on his studies, Freeman
suggests another, perhaps less tangible, factor which he believes
influences mental health – that of the level of integration or
disintegration of a community.

Defining integration

By *integration* Freeman is referring to the degree to which there is an
identifiable and coherent structure within a community to which
groups and individuals may feel themselves to be related. Such a
structure may be focused on an ethnic or religious grouping, or an
occupational grouping, for example, a mining village. He suggests that it is generally believed that a more integrated community promotes mental health, and, interestingly, that mental
health promotes a more integrated community; he points out,
however, that the relationship is not simple.

Defining disintegration

What, then, is *disintegration* and how does it come about? Various
community characteristics have been used to assess disintegration,
including high crime rates, poverty, higher rates of suicide, rapid
cultural change, and fragmented communication patterns. Perhaps more significantly, it has been thought of as an absence
among members of a society of a feeling of affiliation, of
belonging, with shared values and norms becoming weak or
absent. Those living in an area may feel alienated from any
participation in the life of their locality. It is thought such
disintegration results from the rate of social change in a community outstripping the community's ability to adapt to those
changes. In a sense the community has lost its coping mechanisms
or found them inadequate in the face of such great changes.

Housing policy

Two major changes in particular stand out as having a great impact on our cities in recent years, both of which could contribute to disintegration. The first of these is housing policy which has in many towns replaced slum housing with new estates, and in the process may have broken up established communities. Many of those rehoused in the estates of the 1960s have found that the new designs militated against re-establishment of a sense of community. The community architecture movement with its encouragement of current projects to refurbish large inner-city estates on "defensible space" lines – removing communicating walkways and pedestrian through-routes – may be seen as a response to a sense of disintegration.

Mass unemployment

The second more recent change is that of mass unemployment. The development of industrialised, urban societies has led to a huge diversity in the occupations of the members of those societies. Where there is relatively full employment there is, therefore, a degree of interdependence within the community. We need factory workers, doctors, clerks, dustmen, bakers, nurses, teachers, building workers, car mechanics, and an almost infinite number of other workers in a modern city or town – and they all need each other. Such interdependence must, in part, contribute to a more integrated society. However, as unemployment figures have risen the extent of this interdependence has decreased, since there are large numbers of people who cannot easily contribute to society through work. Hence another way in which a society may maintain its integration is eroded.

It would seem, however, that some close-knit communities may survive massive unemployment. A newspaper article describing the old steel town of Consett, where there is now a male unemployment rate of at least 35%, pointed out that there was still a strong sense of community (Chester and Tighe, 1985). Many redundant steelworkers maintained their self-esteem by becoming very involved in improving the appearance of their houses and the neighbourhood, and through weight-training and other sports. In talking about the importance of the now active

Community Programme a local minister said: "Unemployment has an isolating effect. It drives people in on themselves." It appears that strong family and friendship ties have contributed to the maintenance of a close-knit community, where there is no stigma attached to being unemployed. The authors point out, however, that if high levels of unemployment continue the future of Consett could yet be very different.

Another article, this time examining the north-eastern town of Hartlepool which has the highest unemployment rate on the British mainland, found that the *absence* of any housing development over the past decade has lessened the damaging effects of unemployment there (Gregory, 1984). The back-to-back housing contains large networks of extended families that have survived intact and are now flourishing. Within an extended family there is usually one member with a job and a wage, and money and services are shared around. Home and family have become as important to other family members, as they have traditionally been to women, as a place where people are recognised and valued as individuals. A person could be understandably wary about leaving such a supportive, cohesive community in order to find employment elsewhere.

A second way in which unemployment may influence the degree of integration is where the difference in incomes between those in work and those unemployed can lead to widely varying standards of living between different sections of the community. This, too, can contribute to divisions in society.

Characteristics of community life

It would be misleading to claim that the characteristics of community life having a negative impact on mental health are confined to modern urban settings, or that high levels of integration are always beneficial. There is some reason to suggest that societies which are highly integrated and rigidly organised may greatly restrict an individual's choices and prevent personal growth in much the same way that a closed family system does (Freeman, 1984). Many rural communities experience their young people leaving the countryside in order to find the freedom, anonymity and adventure in the city that they cannot find at home.

Clearly, the concepts of social integration, disintegration and rigidity are very difficult to quantify. However this does not mean that we should not be attempting to gain some understanding. The nature of the work of CPNs places them in an ideal situation to get to know a great deal about the characteristics of the local community, and to use that knowledge in their work within it. In addition much that is relevant (for example age distribution, the percentage of people living alone, the amount of mobility, etc.) can be found in census data broken down into information about small geographical areas; this is normally available through the health authority's District Information Officer.

Social Support

In addition to the support gained through family membership, people may often be supported emotionally and psychologically through their own social network. A social network has been described as a "personal community" (Hirsch, 1981), made up of family members, friends, work colleagues, fellow club members and so on, through which our social identities are recognised, supported and strengthened. If people do not share parts of their lives with others their social identities can become tenuous, and their participation in society less meaningful to themselves and others. It has been suggested that many people living in western society will have between 16 and 35 people with whom they have significant contact at any one stage of their lives (Wellman, 1981), although not all these contacts will necessarily be positive. By contrast, people who have or have had a mental health problem may have more limited social networks, with more reliance on family members who may at times be hostile. This may be due to lack of confidence in relating to others, difficulties in the development or maintenance of social skills, a lack of interest or motivation to pursue social contacts, or in some cases difficulty in fully reciprocating in the give and take of friendship. As a result their networks tend to be smaller, with less inter-personal intimacy, than are those of others (Gottlieb, 1983).

As well as considering the size of a network, it can also be helpful to look at its density. A dense social network is one in which all or most of the members will also closely relate to each other, while a loose-knit network will contain members whose only link is with the central person. A dense network will often give more security and support than the latter, but loose-knit networks may allow the individual more opportunities than dense networks for growth and change.

But what is the importance of social support? It is thought to act as a protective buffer between a stressor and an "illness" reaction in the individual. It may also, Gottlieb suggests, have a direct positive effect on a person's mental health, regardless of stressful situations: that is, it may insulate people from the harmful effects of stress. This is not anything very remarkable. If we think of our own lives and the importance of our friends and family we can see that our own social networks play a crucial part in providing support and reinforcing our various social identities. When people are in trouble or worried about something happening in their lives, they will generally turn first to their friends and to informal care-givers, rather than to professionals.

People referred to CPNs, however, may have limited social networks, and as a result little social support. This can be the case both for those already living in the community, and also for hospital residents becoming resettled into housing in the district after many years of hospitalisation. Take the following example:

Mr K, aged 61, first became known to the CPN through her work as a member of a team of different professionals planning a small house in the community, into which a number of ex-hospital residents would move. The team would each take on getting to know different potential residents to discover what their needs really were. The nurse spent quite a lot of time with Mr K but found that her collection of information was extremely slow. Although Mr K was not unapproachable or unwelcoming, he was not very able to talk about what he wanted "outside", and after a fairly short time he did not want to talk any more and would wander away. Mr K had been in this particular hospital for a continuous period of 31 years, and had little memory of any other home. He denied having any friends outside or in the hospital, but after a great deal of time spent unobtrusively watching him, and through finding out more from the hospital staff, the CPN noticed that he often sat near another man at meal-times, and that odd words would pass between them. If either of them were absent, or for some reason had to sit at a different table, both became slightly agitated, and tended to eat less. Recently this other man had been ill with 'flu, and Mr K had stopped going out to the local shops for sweets as he normally did, and had become less interested in going to the industrial therapy workshop.

The CPN discovered that Mr K's friend was from another district and, because of this, it was not planned that they would move together. However, with the nursing staff on the ward, she was able to explain the importance of this relationship to the working-group and after some negotiations with the planning authorities, who had not previously considered such a situation, it was agreed that Mr K and his friend would be able to move into the same house.

Mr K's network, then, was very small and easy to overlook. But what about those already living outside hospital? It is also worth considering alternative ways in which some support may be brought into their lives, by working more with the community than with the individual or family. Caplan (1974) has urged professionals to identify the indigenous patterns of lay support in a community and strengthen these to foster more person-to-person support. Four ways in which this could be done (in addition to strengthening the individual's own network) have been described (Froland *et al.*, 1981).

(1) *Volunteer linking* – where existing support for a particular individual is lacking, using lay helpers for friendship, advocacy and support. This could be invaluable for someone like Mr K in helping him to get to know his new neighbourhood.

(2) *Mutual-aid networks* – bringing together people with common problems, or those facing major changes in their lives which could threaten their mental health.

(3) *Neighbourhood helpers* – strengthening the already existing lay helping system by providing consultation and advice to key individuals or groups.

(4) *Community empowerment* – linking up community leaders to increase their influence to improve services, identify community resources and gaps.

Clearly any such project would require a great deal of very detailed knowledge of the local community. No CPN could embark on such work in isolation. However, in some areas similar work is being done by community workers, who have strong links with official and unofficial networks. Although the role of community workers does not focus exclusively on mental health, they could be an invaluable source of information about the locality, and help in identifying ways in which the lay support networks could be strengthened and used.

To give an example, which fits into the second category above, a group for isolated women on an estate could be set up by, say, a

CPN and a social worker in a local community centre. The workers involved might decide to advertise this group in the community centre, the rent office, local shops, and the nearby health centre. It would strengthen the group considerably if it were also to contain one or two women, possibly introduced by the community worker, who were already involved in the day-to-day life of the area, and who had many contacts. These women would be seen by others as people with whom they could identify, and in time the group might develop its own identity, no longer needing the professionals. Having been involved in attempting to establish a group similar to this in the past, we would suggest that it is extremely important that any workers involved are well known to, and trusted and supported by, the relevant groups in the community, prior to starting the group. The project would then be a genuine response to the needs identified by local people. Such a venture could be extremely worthwhile and rewarding (although never "plain sailing").

All the writers in the field of social support and networks have stressed the need for professionals not to impose their view of what is needed and how care and support should be given, when working with indigenous helpers. The advantages of the informal carers in a community, whether they be shopkeepers, nursery staff, hairdressers, tenants association members, or whoever, is that they are integrated into the culture, and share similar norms and expectations. Some of their value to the community comes from the fact that they are *not* professionals and can meet people on their own terms. They are not seen to be coming from a sometimes bureaucratic and unresponsive organisation. They may well, therefore, be better equipped to assess the needs of people in their patch than are the statutory services.

Froland and his colleagues (1981), in writing about the United States, conclude that professionals do not have a monopoly on caring, and that responsibility and control could be shared by formal and informal helpers to a much greater extent than they have been in the past. However, they point out that this requires that the professional staff develop a sensitivity to the norms of the informal helping systems. It is important that such developments are not proposed as a way of increasing the burden of care taken on by lay helpers. Rather, the care provided by families and friends (in many cases women at home) should be acknowledged and supported in practical ways by the statutory services.

Such an approach may be particularly appropriate when CPN

services, and others in the field of community mental health, are attempting to build a link with ethnic minority groups in their district. In such situations it could be quite fruitless, and potentially seen as insensitive, to endeavour to establish a service without enlisting the active support of those who know the community best and working in partnership with them.

Finally, we suggest that, when forming a link with an informal group or community organisation, it is important to be clear about what are the shared aims. If the intention is to help informal carers in the system to identify those with mental health problems at an earlier stage so that they may be referred to the mental health services, then such an aim could conflict with the alternative aim of strengthening the systems of support within the community so that there is less need for referral to professional services at all. We are not suggesting that these two aims cannot run in parallel, but they should always be clarified to the satisfaction of all the parties involved.

The CPN Working with Groups

How then can CPNs use the inherent social nature of human beings in their work with clients? As already suggested, one possible way is to work with groups of people, rather than individuals. There are three types of groups with which CPNs may become involved: (1) already existing groups which may have no specific mental health interest; (2) already existing groups which have come together to focus on mental health or illness issues; and (3) groups formed by mental health professionals, including CPNs, for a specific purpose. As we shall see each type of group requires a different kind of input from a CPN.

Already existing groups with no mental health interest

People in our society spend much of their lives as members of various groups, be they formal, semi-formal or informal. Of course, many such groups and associations will have been formed to focus on tasks or issues other than mental health. However, they provide a forum within which a CPN may do much useful work in the area of health education and primary prevention. They include:

- those formed for educational purposes, such as schools, adult education classes
- those providing accommodation for vulnerable people, such as hostels for homeless people, residential accommodation for elderly people
- community groups, such as residents associations, tenants groups, community centres
- day centres for elderly people
- groups with a religious focus, such as church groups
- recreational groups, such as Scouts, Guides, youth clubs.

In Chapter 4 we introduced the CPN's role in secondary and tertiary prevention (see Table 4.2, p. 79). The remaining kind of prevention is called primary and refers to the reduction of psychiatric disorder in the population as a whole (Caplan, 1969). Primary prevention is more developed in the area of physical health where there are, in some cases, known and generally agreed causes for a particular illness, for example in the relationship between smoking and lung cancer. A health education campaign would then aim to reduce the overall levels of smoking in the whole population. Supplementing this at the level of the kinds of groups mentioned above, there could be talks giving information and advice on how to stop smoking, or perhaps the formation of support groups of those who wish to stop.

Mental ill-health is, however, almost certainly caused by many different factors, and no single cause has yet been identified as the most important. A further obstacle to mental health education is the fact that many people (including sometimes those who are sufferers) may hold preconceived ideas and prejudices about mental illness, and this can hinder early detection programmes. Such beliefs and ideas would not be held only by single individuals but are likely to reflect the attitudes of the primary groups within that community, for example, the person's family, peer groups, friends at work and so on. There would, therefore, be two main functions of mental health education (Freudenberg, 1979):

- to arouse interest, dispel some of the myths surrounding psychiatric illness, and to begin to change attitudes towards it
- to help people to develop the capacity to lead more satisfying lives, particularly by looking at family life, human relationships, etc.

Mental health education and primary prevention are therefore likely to be most useful if focused at a fairly small group level, covering various different aspects of people's lives – for example, stress, life-events, social support, unemployment, family life-cycle and development, ageing and so on. In some instances CPNs have been invited to group meetings to give a series of talks or lead a number of discussions on such subjects. Sometimes this work may be with groups where a potentially difficult life change is anticipated, for example pre-retirement workshops. In such groups the participants may be particularly open to considering the mental health aspects of their life situation. These groups may also have a social support function, as discussed earlier. In other settings it is likely that at least some of the benefit comes from such topics being raised with people who may never have considered them before. Just as people rarely consider their physical health until they become ill, so do they ignore their mental health, thinking they cannot affect its course.

A CPN's links with such formal and semi-formal groups in the community also give him or her a further opportunity to pick up referrals at an early stage, or to act as consultant to any staff the organisation may have.

Already existing groups concerned with specific mental health issues

These may be local or national campaigning groups, including such organisations as local Associations of Mental Health (MIND groups), or the National Schizophrenia Fellowship. Some of these voluntary organisations also provide important elements in a comprehensive community service, such as group homes, day centres, and advice centres. CPNs may often work closely with the staff and clients of such organisations, perhaps acting as co-therapist of a group, participating in the support team for a group home, or bringing their community mental health expertise to a management committee. A good knowledge of what mental health organisations exist in the area ensures that the CPN can link clients and their families into the most appropriate resource. (The main national organisations are listed in Appendix I.)

Self-help groups

A further type of mental health group comprises those established for self-help. Such groups are made up of members who share a common problem, for example, drug dependence, eating disorders, or depression. Their philosophy is that those who require help may also help others, and by doing this will help themselves. They often work by stressing the normality of their members' problems, spreading information, and setting shared goals (Robinson, 1980). At times it will be necessary for the group to encourage its members to drop their own stigmatising ideas about their problems so that they may share their experiences with others. Some groups, for example Alcoholics Anonymous, have a system of sponsorship of new members whereby an established member takes it upon himself or herself to befriend and support a newcomer.

Some self-help groups have been set up in frustrated reaction to the statutory services, and Robinson points out that they can often be seen as counterbalancing the power of the health professionals. However, many groups do not intend to undermine the role of the established services but see themselves as providing something that the state services cannot. In many instances self-help groups are set up in close cooperation with professionals. For example, a CPN might bring together a number of people referred by general practitioners or health visitors who wish to reduce or stop their reliance on minor tranquilliser medication, but are concerned about withdrawal effects. Such a group may initially benefit from the input of a CPN with knowledge of the medication and the reasons for starting it, but might find after a few meetings that it would be equally or more helpful for them to meet without the CPN. This would not imply any criticism of the nurse, but would be a recognition of the ways in which the strengths of the group members could be mobilised to help each other if there were no professional present.

Groups formed for specific mental health purposes

In these groups, formed by CPNs or others, the CPN takes the role of therapist. The range of possible functions of such groups includes social skills, psychotherapy, relatives' support, social support groups for isolated people or those attending a clinic for depôt medication, and many others. Earlier in this chapter we referred to the importance of primary groups and social support; these support groups can act as primary groups for individuals who would otherwise have little interpersonal contact. Other groups might have a clear health education role – for example, a drinkwatchers' group that would aim to help its members to control their drinking in social situations, or an anxiety management group that would help its members to cope with anxiety-provoking situations. Clearly such groups aim to bring together people with problems and experiences in common. The focus of the group would often be on developing behaviour for the outside world, within the supportive environment of the group sessions. Other groups, for example therapy groups, may attempt to arrive at a heterogeneous membership so that the group resembles a microcosm of the real world. The assumption is that individual change may come about through the person experiencing in the group similar interpersonal issues to those encountered in the outside world.

Lieberman (1980) has described several potentially therapeutic properties of groups which do not exist in one-to-one relationships:

- the capacity of the group to develop cohesiveness, so that members feel they belong, are safe and accepted
- the capacity of the group to control behaviour, and to bring about conformity
- the capacity of the group to define reality for its members, and to help members to understand how others see them
- the capacity of the group to induce and reduce powerful feelings
- the capacity to provide a context for social comparison, so that members may compare their feelings and reactions with those of others.

Clearly some of these properties could also have a negative effect on some people, so that the intensity and orientation of the group must be appropriate to its members. For example, it has been found that disturbed psychotic people may not benefit from a group in which intense feelings could be aroused or interpretations are used, but nevertheless they may be helped by a warm and supportive rehabilitation group. Such a group could provide quite isolated and socially unskilled people with an opportunity to form friendships, and to increase their competence in dealing with others in a safe, non-threatening setting. Group membership encourages the clients to communicate with each other and to share their feelings and experiences with others apart from professionals. In addition, group meetings give the CPN an opportunity to observe how the members behave in social situations, and may in some instances lessen the possibility of the client developing dependence on the nurse.

The Nurse as Client's Advocate

Much has recently been written or spoken about the role of the nurse as the patient's or client's advocate. It has perhaps become fashionable for nurses to claim that they have incorporated the advocacy role into their overall work, or to say that they as nurses have been doing it all along. But what is meant by advocacy, and do CPNs have a part to play? An advocate has been described as: "a person who effectively represents, as if they were his own, the interests of a mentally ill or mentally handicapped person who has major needs which are unmet, and likely to remain unmet, without special intervention" (Gostin, 1984, p. 5).

Advocates provide friendship, protection and representation, and through these help to improve the individual's quality of life, and his or her access to services. They are also concerned with the person's right to respect, dignity and privacy. Advocacy is fundamentally about the conviction that people with mental illness or handicap have a right to all the services received by others, and to special services related to any special needs they may have. There have been several schemes in hospitals for mentally handicapped people in which independent volunteers have befriended residents and taken on acting as their advocates to the hospital authorities (Sang and O'Brien, 1984). Such a role can in some cases lead to some conflict with the professionals involved. If, in other situations, the advocate were a member of health authority staff there could be a conflict of interests and divided loyalties. This has been one of the reasons cited for the difficulty of nurses taking on a full advocacy role. Nevertheless Gostin points out that the input of nurses is still extremely valuable.

What, then, does advocacy entail for the community psychiatric nurse? Another definition, coined this time by a nurse, says "advocacy is a means of transferring power back to the patient to enable him to control his own affairs" (Walsh, 1985, p. 24). This is certainly what community psychiatric nursing is, or should be, about. However, in its pure form advocacy is said to require independence from the service, a long-term commitment to a small number of people, and training. Not all of these conditions can readily be met by CPNs, yet there are elements of the philosophy of advocacy upon which CPNs may draw. Four main issues have been highlighted (Brown, 1985):

- the quality of care a patient or client receives
- access to care
- that a patient or client should be fully informed about the care offered and received
- awareness of alternatives to the care.

These are all areas in which CPNs may become involved, and indeed many are already doing so. For example, there has been recent publicity on possible long-term brain damage caused by major tranquillisers. Some CPNs have responded by updating themselves on the relevant pharmacological information, and discussing the issue with prescribing medical staff, so that they are better equipped to help clients in the choices they make. Such action addresses at least the last two of Brown's advocacy issues.

Elsewhere CPNs are also becoming involved in acting on behalf of clients and representing them to other authorities, for example, social security offices, or housing departments. In other situations, the nurse may act as an intermediary between a client and the wider society, for example by meeting the neighbours of a newly converted group home, and subsequently facilitating the house residents to do likewise. Such work will, in many cases, lead on to encouraging and helping the client to represent himself or herself to these agencies or groups, with the support of the nurse in the background if necessary.

Clearly, if there is progress in the direction of clients having more information about the treatment they receive, and they are able to make more informed choices based on some knowledge of alternatives, there will inevitably be some transfer of power to the patients of the kind Walsh is suggesting.

The Welfare State and Mental Health

We have discussed in earlier sections of this book the way in which the meeting of several basic needs – for example, shelter, food, warmth and so on – may contribute to an individual's mental health. Clearly government policy, and in particular the welfare state, plays an important part, directly or indirectly, in addressing some of these needs. Since issues such as benefits or housing impinge so strongly on the lives of CPNs' clients it is very helpful for CPNs to have some understanding of the systems involved. Regulations do, of course, change from time to time. Up-to-date information and advice may be obtained through DHSS offices, housing offices, citizens' advice bureaux etc.

State benefits

The system of state benefits is extremely complex and CPNs cannot be expected to have a grasp of all the details. There will also be some major changes to the benefits system in 1988 following the 1985 social security review. Therefore, we intend to highlight the main benefits of current importance for people with mental health problems. (There is now a microcomputer program that will give advice on an individual's benefit entitlement if certain information is fed in. This could be used in future by CPN services with access to a microcomputer.) Some benefits are paid only to those who have, through previous employment, paid the necessary amount of national insurance contributions in the relevant part of the year; these benefits include: sickness, maternity, unemployment, retirement, and widow's.

Other benefits, probably more commonly claimed by people seen by CPNs, are given to everyone who is entitled, irrespective of their contributions; these include:

● child benefit
● supplementary benefit – paid to those who are unemployed (but receiving no unemployment benefit or a small amount), retired (on a pension not adequate to their needs), or in low-paid part-time employment; in 1988 this will be replaced by the "income support scheme" and a "social fund" to cover discretionary payments.

Supplementary benefit

Supplementary benefit is normally made up of an allowance for the person and any dependents, and any "additional requirements" benefit, which can cover special diets, laundry (if all residents of the household are ill or infirm, or there is more washing than normal, for example, if someone is incontinent), blindness, extra baths needed for medical reasons, and so on. If a person is receiving supplementary benefit he or she also has a right to free:

- national health service dental treatment
- national health service glasses
- national health service prescriptions
- school meals.

It is now known that large numbers of people entitled to supplementary benefit either do not claim their full entitlement, or make no claim at all, for various reasons including lack of information, the feeling of accepting charity, and the possible stigma attached. CPNs and their colleagues working in the community are well-placed to dispel these ideas and to encourage those with whom they come in contact to make full claims.

Attendance allowance

There are also some other benefits for which some CPN clients may be eligible, for example attendance allowance. This allowance is payable to someone who is severely disabled, either physically or mentally, and who requires frequent attention in connection with eating, drinking, keeping clean and warm, and walking, or continual supervision to avoid danger to self or others. There are two rates, a lower one for someone who needs such attention during either day or night, and a higher rate for someone who needs attention during both day and night. In both cases the individual must have required such care for at least 6 months before being entitled to the allowance. Attendance allowance is not means-tested, and, unlike some of the other benefits, it is normally paid in full on top of any other benefits the person may receive. Many CPN clients, particularly elderly people, could be eligible for such a benefit, but may be unaware of its existence or of how to apply.

Invalid care allowance (ICA)

It is also possible for the person caring for someone who receives attendance allowance to claim invalid care allowance (ICA). While attendance allowance is for the person who requires the care, invalid care allowance is paid to the carer, who must spend at least 35 hours a week caring for the disabled person, and must not earn more than a specified amount in other employment. At present it is not payable to married women who are living with their husbands, even if the person for whom they are caring is not their husband. (This restriction is currently being contested in the courts, and a welfare adviser has advised all married women who would qualify for ICA if they were not married to make a claim; see Graham, 1985.) In addition, ICA will not be paid if the person is receiving the same amount or more of other benefits, including supplementary benefit.

Information leaflets about these and other benefits and application forms are available from DHSS offices and Citizens' Advice Bureaux. In addition, each year the Child Poverty Action Group issues its *National Welfare Benefits Handbook*, which gives detailed information about supplementary benefit, family income supplement (to be replaced in 1987 by family credit benefit which will give more support to the lowest paid and less to those with a slightly higher income), housing benefits and health benefits.

Housing

Shelter is one of the most fundamental requirements of human beings, involving as it does (or should do) warmth, protection from the elements, and safety and sanctuary from the outside world. In the United Kingdom there are three main sectors of housing; owner occupied, privately rented and local authority provided. The first of these has expanded in recent decades as more people are buying their own homes. Privately rented housing is becoming less common, while local authority rented accommodation is expanding fairly slowly (Gaffin, 1981). The range of the quality of housing is enormous, but generally it is thought that the worst conditions are likely to be found in the privately rented sector, and as a result this is where some of the more vulnerable members of society live.

Local authorities tend to give priority to certain groups of people, including those with children, ill or disabled, or elderly people. These priorities are also laid down in the Housing (Homeless Persons) Act of 1977. It is extremely beneficial for CPNs to have some knowledge of the provisions of this particular act, since they may find some clients affected by it. The Act covers people who are homeless or threatened with homelessness within the next 28 days, and who also fit into one of the following categories:

- the person with dependent children
- the person whose homelessness has been caused by a flood, fire or other emergency
- the person, or someone who lives with him or her, who is "vulnerable" as a result of old age, mental illness or handicap, physical disability, etc.

If a person fits these criteria he or she, plus members of the household, must be rehoused by the local authority. However, if the local authority has little or no vacant housing it is likely to place families in temporary accommodation, such as short-life housing or bed and breakfast hotels, which in some areas may last for months or years. This is especially likely in inner-city areas. In addition, the local authority is not obliged to find permanent housing for people who are deemed to have made themselves homeless intentionally, even if they fit all the other criteria. In these circumstances the authority should provide temporary accommodation and housing advice.

The significance of this Act to CPNs is that any homeless person, whether single or not, who is vulnerable as a result of illness, including mental illness, must be treated as a priority for housing by the local authority. People who are going to be discharged from hospital within a month should also be considered as being threatened with homelessness.

Some people who are discharged from hospital, particularly those who need ongoing rehabilitation after a lengthy admission or who have for some other reason become homeless, may be considered for hostel or group home accommodation. This is usually provided by local authorities or voluntary organisations, but some health authorities, for example Oxford, now have a number of group homes in which CPNs are closely involved (Leopoldt, 1980). Several other health authorities are developing hostels staffed by nurses as one element in their comprehensive community services.

Occupation

In Chapter 2 we discussed some of the many benefits that people may derive from employment and the potentially damaging effects of unemployment. For those who have, or have had, a mental health problem the effects of unemployment may be compounded. At a time of high unemployment those who have had an episode of illness may have great difficulty in finding work, perhaps because of the reluctance of employers to take them on. There are unfortunately still many generalised misconceptions about the effects of mental ill-health on a person's ability to work. Some people, of course, may not be able to pick up their previous occupation, and may feel instead that they would like to do something less demanding or stressful. However, provided that a realistic assessment of their skills is made it is likely that they could cope with the right kind of alternative work. While some people may have difficulty finding work, others may have a series of jobs that they are unable to keep. Both of these situations can be extremely distressing and demoralising. It could therefore be very beneficial for the CPN to involve specialist workers in this field with a client who wishes to pursue employment and who is having such difficulties.

Disablement Resettlement Officers (DROs) are specially trained members of staff, normally based in job centres, who aim to help find suitable employment for anyone who has been ill or is disabled. They work with people who have both physical illness or disability, and those with mental ill-health. DROs will usually have contact with local companies and can use these contacts to put job-hunters in touch with potential employers. They will also have information about any retraining courses which could be appropriate. Many DROs may, however, have fairly limited experience or training in the employment of people with mental health problems. They may therefore greatly value a link with, and the opinions of, mental health professionals. It can also be extremely valuable for mental health workers to provide some continuing support to clients who have gone back into open employment, perhaps after a lengthy absence. In some instances this could entail visiting the client at his or her place of work, or liaising with the employer who may be unsure how best to help. Such support may be particularly valuable in the first months of a new job.

If open employment is not possible there are other options in some areas. Some voluntary organisations are developing sheltered workshop projects, some of which can take clients for up to one or two years. Such projects aim to build up a person's confidence and basic work skills, as well as to provide particular training in, for example, clerical skills, typing, printing, or working in a shop. Gloag (1985) has listed a number of other types of occupational opportunities for people who have had physical or mental ill-health, including:

- *Employment rehabilitation centres* (run by the Manpower Services Commission) offer courses of six weeks or longer, for assessment, occupational guidance, and work practice; at the end they may recommend a particular training course.
- *Job rehearsal*, following an ERC course, giving up to three weeks experience in open employment, with allowances paid by the MSC.
- *Job introduction* – a trial period of up to six weeks during which the MSC pays the employer a subsidy towards the person's wages; at the end of the period the person is employed if suitable.
- *Sheltered placement schemes* – allowing one or more people with a psychiatric problem to work in open employment; the person is employed and paid by a sponsoring organisation (for example, a voluntary body or local authority) which is then reimbursed by the employer for the work actually done.

Gloag (1985) makes the point that what is needed is a range of workshops and activity centres with differing levels of demands placed on clients. It appears that a supportive environment that allows clients to succeed rather than reaffirms their previous failure is also very important. Unfortunately in many areas places in employment rehabilitation services are still rather limited.

Summary

This chapter has examined the relationship between the individual and the wider social system, and the implications of this for the work of the CPN. All of us are members of primary groups in addition to our families, and we live for longer or shorter periods of time in localities with varying degrees of a sense of community. Social changes within such localities and society generally (for example housing development, unemployment) have an impact on such a sense of community and on those who live there. Following this we discussed the social support that a person can gain from others, and the need for CPNs to recognise the importance of this.

In considering the individual within the wider society we then went on to look at the CPN's role in working with groups and in taking on an advocacy role on behalf of clients. The final section referred to some of the main social policy issues – state benefits, housing, employment – that have a bearing on those who have mental health problems, and consequently on the work of CPNs. In the next chapter we consider how the CPN fits into her or his own system.

References

Brown, M. (1985) Matter of commitment. *Nursing Times*, **1 May,** 26–7.

Caplan, G. (1969) *An Approach to Community Mental Health.* Tavistock, London.

Caplan, G. (1974) Support systems, in Caplan, G. (ed.) *Support Systems and Community Mental Health.* Basic Books, New York.

Chester, L. and Tighe, C. (1985) Consett has seen its future – and it's workless. *Sunday Times Magazine*, **15 September,** 24–32.

Freeman, H. L. (1984) Introduction, in Freeman, H. L. (ed.) *Mental Health and the Environment.* Churchill Livingstone, London.

Freudenberg, R. K. (1979) Mental health education, in Sutherland, I. (ed.) *Health Education.* George Allen and Unwin, London.

Froland, C. *et al.* (1981) Linking formal and informal support systems, in Gottlieb, B. H. (ed.) *Social Networks and Social Support.* Sage Publications, Beverly Hills.

Gaffin, J. (ed.) (1981) *The Nurse and the Welfare State.* HM & M Publishers, Aylesbury.

Gloag, D. (1985) Occupational rehabilitation and return to work: 2 – psychiatric disability. *British Medical Journal,* **290,** 1201–3.

Gostin, L. (1984) Foreword, in Sang, B. and O'Brien, J. (eds.). *Advocacy – the UK and the American Experience.* King Edward's Hospital Fund for London, London.

Gottlieb, B. H. (1983) *Social Support Strategies.* Sage Publications, London.

Graham, A. (1985) Defying the directive. *Nursing Times – Community Outlook*, **June,** 11.

Gregory, P. (1984) You don't heave a brick through your uncle's window. *Guardian*, **18 February,** 7.

Hirsch, B. J. (1981) Social networks and the coping process, in Gottlieb, B. H. (ed.). *Social Networks and Social Support.* Sage Publications, Beverly Hills.

Leopoldt, H. (1980) The psychiatric group home – 2. *Nursing Times*, **15 May,** 866–8.

Lieberman, M. A. (1980) Group methods, in Kanfer, F. H. and Goldstein, A. P. (eds). *Helping People Change.* Pergamon Press, New York.

Pons, V. (1977) Communities and cities, in Worsley, P. (ed.) *Introducing Sociology.* Penguin, Harmondsworth.

Robinson, D. (1980) Self-help health groups, in Smith, P. (ed.) *Small Groups and Personal Change*. Methuen, London.

Sang, B. and O'Brien, J. (1984). *Advocacy – the UK and the American Experience*. King Edwards Hospital Fund for London, London.

Sprott, W. J. H. (1958) *Human Groups*. Penguin, Harmondsworth.

Walsh, P. (1985) Speaking up for the patient, *Nursing Times*, **1 May,** 24–6.

Wellman, B. (1981) Applying network analysis to the study of support, in Gottlieb, B. H. (ed.). *Social Networks and Social Support*. Sage Publications, Beverly Hills.

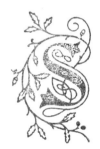

6

The CPN's System

In the previous two chapters we have discussed the individual as a member of different systems, first the immediate family, and second the community and wider society. In this chapter we shall continue this theme by considering the system or systems within which the CPN operates, and examining how the different and sometimes interrelated elements within these systems affect her or his work.

The CPN Team

The CPN's immediate, local system is the CPN team. Although many CPNs may spend much of their working week on their own, they will generally be members of a team which meets up on a regular basis, to discuss business, clinical and policy matters, for supervision, or for training and education.

We saw in Chapter 3 that there is wide variation in the way in which CPN services are organised. We pointed out several factors that have a particular influence on this, including the location and type of CPN bases, whether there is an open or closed referral system, and the number, grades and any specialisation of CPNs employed. At present the largest single grade employed in CPN services is sister/charge nurse II. This would seem to reflect a recognition of the fairly independent and autonomous way in which most CPNs work. However, it may become desirable in the future to establish nursing teams made up of different grades. Such teams could be responsible for a larger number of clients than would ordinarily be on a single charge nurse's caseload. Staff nurses in such teams could be in training posts with consequently less responsibility, while nursing assistants could take on some other tasks, for example, helping with daily living skills like shopping, cooking, hygiene etc. which could greatly extend the community psychiatric nursing service provided to clients.

Other practical matters also affect the operation of a service, such as the availability of secretarial staff to carry out typing and reception duties, and to take accurate messages from the many people who try to contact CPNs by telephone; or regular and unproblematic access to a room large enough to hold all the members of a particular service and their students and visitors.

The management structure and philosophy can also, of course, make an impact on the ways in which a CPN service operates. The research carried out by Skidmore and Friend (1984) on 120 CPNs in 12 different services found that 60% of the nurses in their study visited almost exactly eight clients a day. They discovered that this figure had been defined as an appropriate workload by managers who were used to an institutional setting and not familiar with the work of CPNs. In addition to prescribing the number of visits to be made, some of these managers appeared to expect staff to clock on and off at the beginning and end of the day. Many of the nurses resented this, feeling that their management had little concept of what they did, and in some cases they complied with "an attitude of passive hostility", and reduced the amount of work they did. Most of the nurses within such structures felt that they would contribute more to their work if they had more "enlightened" management, ideally someone who had experience of being a CPN and possibly still carried a small caseload.

A case has also been put forward for the further creation of clinical senior nurses in CPN services. Although, by contrast, these would probably not be line management posts they would clearly have an important part to play in influencing the philosophy and approach of a team. Manchester (1985) has suggested three main roles: consultation and advice; education and training; and clinical. The senior nurses would retain their clinical credibility by maintaining a small caseload and being actively involved in the work of their charge nurse colleagues. A very similar model operates in some health districts where there are team leader/ senior nurse posts. Again these senior nurses may not be line managers, but they nevertheless have a responsibility for monitoring and coordinating a team of, say, six or seven CPNs, providing or enabling supervision, maintaining a high standard of care, and carrying out day-to-day management of the team.

A further, very important factor that influences the *modus operandi* of a CPN service is the degree to which there is a generally recognised and agreed framework or strategy within which the service can determine future developments and review progress. We saw in Chapter 3 that the growth and development of CPN services have been generally fairly *ad hoc*, until very recently. As services become larger, and there is increasing realisation that they must attempt to meet the needs of their particular districts, the importance of a plan which is closely related to the district's overall strategy for mental health services becomes clearer. Such a strategy could be drafted, discussed and revised by members of the CPN service, and would provide a clear statement on a number of issues, for example:

- the basic principles underpinning the service, including accessibility, localness, attempting to meet the needs of all people with mental health problems, etc.
- the way in which it is envisaged that the particular CPN service would develop further, for example, as a generic service but containing some people with special expertise, and as a service working closely with both psychiatric services and primary health care
- the main areas of responsibility of the service with reference to hospital closures
- future grades of staff and possible hours of working.

Perhaps most importantly such a plan should have the agreement of all the members of the CPN service, having been fully discussed and amended by them. It need not simply be an academic exercise, but a working document, which would be referred to often and revised from time to time. (An example of a strategy document is given in Appendix II.)

CPNs and Stress

Much of a CPN's work is carried out alone, or on territory that is perhaps unfamiliar and over which she has no control. In addition, CPNs are constantly meeting new people, many of whom may be feeling frightened, anxious, bewildered or occasionally hostile. It is a job placing many demands on its practitioners. Some of these demands will be among the reasons for people wishing to take up, and stay in, nursing in general, and community psychiatric nursing in particular. However, when demands become threatening rather than challenging they contribute to stress, and the nurse may find it difficult to cope. In recent years nursing in general has been identified as a potentially stressful occupation, but particularly so in those areas of nursing which are more likely to involve two-way relationships and more sharing (for example, psychiatric nursing) rather than more technical procedures (Firth, 1984).

In hospital settings the old methods of organising nursing care by task allocation prevented nurses from becoming particularly involved in the lives of their individual patients. The resulting distancing from patients could act as a protective mechanism against the stress potentially caused by the responsibility of caring for another person, and attempting to meet his or her needs (Menzies, 1960). With the introduction of individual patient care, and a holistic approach to nursing care planning, some concern has been expressed that without greater support and appropriate training nurses could experience even higher levels of stress (Hancock, 1984). Hancock also points out that nurses working in the community have by definition almost always had an individual, continuing and intimate relationship with their patients or clients and their families, and this brings with it similar pressures. They may have already been experiencing the strains that hospital nurses are feeling now.

Stress is a topic that is also being investigated in fields outside nursing, and some writers have tried to identify general factors that could contribute to it. Fingret (1985), in defining it as "an excess of environmental demands over the individual's capability to meet them", gave a list of such factors which included:

(1) *Work underload* (not a problem for most CPNs!)
(2) *Work overload* – both quantitative and qualitative (for example, being asked to take on work that is beyond the CPN's level of skill); this can lead to job dissatisfaction and lowered self-esteem.
(3) *Role ambiguity* and a lack of clarity about objectives, colleagues' expectations and the scope of the job; again, this could be relevant to CPNs whose jobs may often be relatively undefined.
(4) *Role conflict* – conflicting demands arising from different elements of the work, or from clients, nursing management

and colleagues with whom the CPN has links (for example, respecting a client's wish in refusing medication when the prescribing general practitioner has specifically asked that he should be encouraged to have it).

(5) *Responsibility for people* – generally more stressful than responsibility for things; this clearly applies to all nursing and other caring professions.

(6) *Lack of opportunities* for career development.

(7) *Competing commitments* between home and work, and major life-events in the individual's personal life which could affect the capacity to handle demands at work.

(8) *Change* – for example, reorganisation, relocation, major changes in policies.

In considering such a list it is apparent that the life of a CPN could, therefore, be quite stressful. But how would we recognise stress in ourselves or others? Some people might find they have physical symptoms including headaches, upset stomach, increased muscle tension, increased smoking (still very common among nurses). Others experience psychological effects such as a negative self-image, feelings of powerlessness, a decrease in job satisfaction, irritability, a deterioration in quality of care, a tendency to blame others for things going wrong. When stress is prolonged and unrelenting it may lead to what has been called "burn-out", manifested by many different indices including chronic fatigue, anger, depression, loss of sympathy, interpersonal conflict with colleagues, disregarding high priority tasks, negative or cynical attitudes about clients, and withdrawal from day-to-day work (see McCarthy, 1985).

Support and supervision

How, then, can such a state of affairs be prevented? The answer, in part at least, seems to be through systems of support and supervision. Clients may gain support in a multitude of ways (see Chapter 5) and, of course, this also is true for CPNs, who will certainly vary considerably in their responses to stress, depending on their basic personality, previous experiences, and coping skills. Support may be found amongst peers, colleagues outside nursing, senior nurses, and in the CPNs' private lives. Hancock (1984) outlines four main roles for senior nurses in this respect:

● support for clinical nurses, including when things go wrong

- providing nursing leadership
- putting the nursing view to others
- enabling peer group support and meetings

An interesting small-scale study has been reported in which nurses were interviewed to find out in what ways they felt they needed support (Firth, 1984). The nurses worked in a medical ward for elderly people, but the findings are relevant in a wider context. The most common response was that they felt they needed a number of things which Firth bracketed together and called emotional support, including being listened to, receiving praise, reassurance and feedback, feeling understood, being consulted. The availability and approachability of senior staff were very important. Practical action although helpful was not seen as providing as much as good communication and emotional support. Firth concludes by making the point that staff who feel unsupported cannot help others and the problem can spread throughout a unit or team, resulting in low morale, high absenteeism and so on.

There are, in addition, more planned ways in which senior staff can support nurses, for example through the monitoring and reviewing of workloads, career development and supervision. The first of these demonstrates that the senior member of staff has a genuine concern that the workload is manageable for that CPN, that it does not overstretch her in terms of the actual amount of work, or in terms of the demands it places on her skills, and that she has a mix of clients requiring a range of types of contact and intervention. Many of the factors given earlier, described as stressors by Fingret, can be identified, considered and hopefully modified in such review sessions. For example, not uncommonly a fairly new member of staff may feel very anxious about the lack of clear direction in how to go about developing her role. Fingret would call this lack of direction "role ambiguity". Once picked up the CPN's anxiety could be relieved by the joint devising of an action plan which would clarify the main objectives and the steps to be taken. Similarly, Hancock stresses the need for new members of staff to know what is expected of them, and to be able to identify one member of staff who will be friendly and supportive. It is possible that, in our desire for CPN services to determine their own direction, we have overlooked some of the needs of newer members of staff.

Other features of the work setting can affect the extent to

which someone will feel satisfied with their job, including opportunities for promotion, post-basic education and training courses, and part-time working and job-sharing (without loss of promotion prospects). These and other issues related to career development may be raised in the context of a general review. For example, in order not to lose very experienced CPNs who wish to go part-time to raise a family, it could be helpful to investigate instead ways in which two CPNs could actively share a caseload, working part of the week each (job-sharing either formally or informally). In this way clients would, it is hoped, continue to receive the same standard of care and the part-time staff would generally feel less isolated from their full-time colleagues.

Workload monitoring and review are sometimes seen to overlap with supervision, although the latter is often used to describe time in which particular clients and families on a CPN's caseload are focused on in more depth. Because of the isolated nature of much of a CPN's work it is particularly important that all nurses have access to supervision on a regular basis. This can take place in a number of ways, in individual sessions with a senior nurse, a colleague from another discipline, or another member of the CPN team, or in a peer group setting (with or without an outside supervisor). Which supervision arrangement is used will depend on the type of client being discussed, the preferred way of working of CPN and supervisor, and whether any specialised input is required. For example, a CPN may seek supervision from a psychotherapist or family therapist for her work with specific clients.

There are both advantages and disadvantages to individual and group supervision. In individual sessions there is an opportunity for a close, trusting relationship to develop, and for a greater amount of time to be spent discussing particular clients. In group sessions members may learn a great deal from each other, so that the confidence of other group members is enhanced. In addition, in such a setting the work of CPNs becomes more visible to their peers than it is normally. This can be potentially threatening to some people, but it can also result in very helpful feedback.

The aim of supervision sessions is to facilitate the nurse in developing a different perspective on her work with clients, by encouraging greater self-awareness and building on her strengths and therapeutic and coping skills. As a process effective supervision is educative without being didactic, since it promotes learning, and increases confidence and problem-solving skills in a supportive setting, but does not generally issue instructions or direct the CPN's work. There are several requirements for it to work well. It needs to be recognised as valuable to those taking part and to their managers, and as a consequence of this it needs to be a regular commitment, which does not get eroded by other demands on the CPN's or the supervisor's time. It should also be seen as important not just for relatively inexperienced members of staff, but for all staff. The self-awareness that can arise through supervision is not once-and-for-all but a continuing process. The responsibility for facilitating supervision for all members of a CPN team, and in some cases for providing it, fits well with the role of senior nurse or team leader in the service.

It would be misleading to imply that systems of supervision and workload monitoring only benefit individual CPNs. They can also be extremely important for the service in providing a forum for examining the degree of fit between the direction in which a CPN's work is going and the overall strategy for the development of the service as a whole.

The Wider System Surrounding the CPN

While the team is generally the most immediate local system for the CPN, there will also be a wider system within which he or she operates, made up of a large variety of different disciplines and agencies. The provision of a community mental health service is now often thought of as a complex joint venture involving the psychiatric and primary health care services of health authorities, the social services of local authorities, and numerous local voluntary associations. The work of CPNs will almost certainly bring them into contact with all of these agencies. It may therefore be helpful to consider each of them separately.

The psychiatric services

Historically, this has been the most important link for many CPN services, developing as they have done on the same site as the psychiatric hospital. Some services, however, have grown up quite independently from psychiatric services, under the auspices of primary health care provision. Others have since moved away from hospital bases and put energy into working almost exclusively in primary health care settings. In some districts this different approach is reflected in the management structure, with CPNs being managed by community services rather than mental health services. The disadvantage of not having well-established links with in-patient, day-patient and out-patient facilities is that CPN teams could lose their availability to those people who are already using such psychiatric provision (McKendrick, 1984b).

CPNs are actually in an excellent position to act as a link between hospital and the community, both in terms of facilitating effective discharge from hospital or, in some instances, easing a person's admission. Such work, however, requires regular input, communication and commitment on the part of the CPN and the ward team. A CPN linked to a particular ward team could attend meetings regularly with ward staff, and take on an active role as a member of that team. In this way planning for discharge could involve the input of the CPN from the earliest possible stage, rather than the referral to the CPN service being made just prior to the person going home. As we saw in Chapter 3, Goldberg (1985) has suggested that such active involvement of CPNs could shorten the length of admission for many patients. CPNs also have a great deal to contribute to the information available to the ward team, through their knowledge of the community from which the in-patients come. This may be particularly valuable where the psychiatric hospital is geographically removed from its catchment area. We are not, however, prescribing regular attendance at all ward rounds, since this may not always be relevant to the CPN. Rather we suggest that the CPN and the ward team should negotiate how best the link can be established and maintained. This could be done in a number of ways.

Some districts are now developing nursing posts to do outreach work from a ward base and of course other disciplines, including psychiatrists, psychologists, occupational therapists and hospital-based social workers, often spend some of their time working in the community. In some districts this is much more advanced than in others, but it is certainly going to become more common practice everywhere. Rather than setting up totally separate systems it makes sense for such staff to work closely with nurses already well experienced in working in the community. CPN services may gradually become integrated into multidisciplinary community teams. (This is discussed more fully in Chapter 7.)

Another important potential function of CPNs relates to hospital closure policies. As many districts are developing plans to bring long-stay hospital residents back to live in smaller local psychiatric units, hostels, or group homes, CPNs can contribute a considerable amount to planning groups about the local community and the facilities available. They may also (as we discussed in earlier chapters) take on an active rehabilitative role with clients who are discharged into completely or relatively unstaffed accommodation. At present this is a fairly undeveloped area of CPN work. We suggest that it may not easily combine with the more established role of CPNs, since it requires different patterns of working and smaller caseloads. It should still nevertheless be seen as an area of need for which CPN services have a responsibility. This may be an area in which we can learn something from our Italian counterparts. (For a fuller discussion see Brooker, 1985).

Primary health care services

The 1985 CPNA Survey found that there is a wide range in the number of CPNs based in health centres or general practitioner practices, from 1.5% in Yorkshire to 43.5% in Northern Ireland. In addition to those CPNs who have their main base in a primary health care facility there are also many CPNs who have established links with the staff of health centres and clinics, take referrals from them, and work closely with them. The CPN's role in primary health care is, therefore, now well recognised in many districts. The subject of CPN bases has been fully discussed in general and policy terms in Chapter 3. We shall therefore now concentrate on the impact of links with primary health care services on the work of the individual CPN.

General practitioners

It is known that a significant proportion of people consulting their general practitioners have a mental health problem, although this may often be poorly defined (Robertson and Scott, 1985). As community care develops and fewer people remain in hospital, the involvement of general practitioners in psychiatric care may increase. Many general practitioners may feel poorly equipped or too busy to treat mental health problems as well as they would like, and find that a number of those they refer to the local psychiatric out-patient department do not attend. In addition it has been reported that general practitioners may under-diagnose certain problems in their patients including chronic alcoholism and senile disorders (Brook and Cooper, 1975). The availability of a nurse who is able to respond fairly quickly, and can visit a person at home or see him or her in the local health centre has proved to be a big advantage. One survey of general practitioners found that 84% of respondents wished to have a CPN attachment to assist them in assessing and treating psychiatrically ill people in the local community (Sharpe, 1982).

The purpose of primary health care attachments is to make the service available to a larger number of potential clients in a relatively familiar environment. Other mental health professionals, including psychiatrists in some areas, are also forging links with general practitioners. Those studies that have reported on the work of CPNs who are based in health centres suggest that, at present, the clients referred to them may be quite different from those coming from psychiatric agencies. For example, Robertson and Scott (1985) report that 82% of all referrals to the health centre-based CPNs were from general practitioners, and were often people with no previous psychiatric history. They used a list of presenting problems grouped into:

- problems of mood and affect
- problems of thinking
- problems with social environment
- behavioural problems
- physical symptoms.

They found that the most common problems were those of mood or affect, followed by behavioural problems (often alcohol) and social problems. Contact was often short. The authors conclude that the system of easy access to the CPNs removed the potential stigma of a psychiatric label for some clients by preventing the need for psychiatric referral. However, we must be cautious in making such claims. Another report on the same scheme points out that prior to the input to a particular health centre of a small multidisciplinary mental health team (which included a CPN) the number of referrals from the health centre to hospital psychiatrists was around 20 per year (Corser and Ryce, 1977). Immediately, referrals to the team went up to double this figure and then continued to rise each following year. This would suggest that the mental health team were seeing a rather different group of clients in addition to those who would otherwise be referred to traditional psychiatric services.

Another study examined the work of five CPNs attached to 30 GPs in Northamptonshire, with a brief to work with elderly people (Tough, Kingerlee and Elliott, 1980). The researchers found that approximately half the people referred had depression, and just over a quarter had a diagnosis of dementia. They commented on the fact that although the CPNs had many elderly clients they provided little or no physical nursing care. As a result some elderly people may have had two or more professionals coming into their homes for different purposes, possibly exacerbating any confusion they may have had. Despite this reservation, the authors felt this was a useful development and commented that the CPNs were well integrated into the primary care teams. The East Dorset Extended Care Project has attempted to overcome the problem of two nursing teams providing care for elderly, frail mentally ill people by employing unqualified patients' aides (Hicks, 1984). The aides work under the guidance and supervision of CPNs and carry out basic, practical tasks, including helping an old person to get up, to dress, wash or bath, or collect their pensions. Because they are involved with only a small number of clients they can visit every day if necessary, and as a result they often become a supportive link for any family carers involved.

Clearly, the success of a CPN attachment to a general practitioner practice or health centre will depend very much on the relationships that exist between the people involved. Community staff are much more likely to refer to a CPN if they know the nurse fairly well, and understand the nature and scope of her work. White (1986) has suggested that an individually negotiated relationship between a CPN and a general practitioner is the most important factor in affecting the number and appropriateness of referrals. A similar finding has also been reported by social workers attached to primary health care teams from their local social services department (Winny and Rushton, 1981). It is therefore important that if a CPN service wishes to receive referrals from general practitioners personal contact is made and if possible maintained with all the general practitioners in the district. By linking CPNs only to well-staffed health centres and large group practices, there is a danger of denying such good access to those general practitioners who work single-handedly, and also of course to people who may need the service but who are not registered with a general practitioner.

Other community nursing services

So far, we have only discussed the CPN's relationship with general practitioners. However, it is also important that there are links with the other community nursing services – health visitors, district nurses and school nurses. (At present approximately half of all CPN services accept nurse-to-nurse referrals but in practice only around 5% of all referrals come from this source.) Such links also create opportunities for nurses to take on a consultative role with each other. For example, a CPN could be consulted by a district nurse who may not wish to make a formal referral but would value the opportunity to talk over a family or an elderly person causing her concern. Similarly the CPN may discuss with a district nurse the nursing care needed by one of her other clients who has a physical illness, or talk over with a health visitor the health educational needs of a family with school-age children.

By establishing such links with all other workers in primary health care, genuine teamwork can be developed. A range of skills can then be provided to meet the varying needs of clients and families without making possibly complex referrals to other agencies or departments. The primary health care team is often described as being made up of a number of general practitioners (Brook and Cooper (1975) suggest five or six), receptionists, attached district nurses, and health visitors. Sometimes CPNs and/or social workers are seen as associate members, at other times they are considered to be core members. In almost all multidisciplinary teams, whether in a hospital or community setting, various issues arise including the team members' conceptions of each others' roles, skills and responsibilities, and the potential overlapping of roles. Clearly all the members of a primary care team will come into contact with people with mental ill-health, and possibly associated social problems, in the course of their work. The potential for role overlap, professional rivalry and misunderstandings between colleagues is therefore great.

These issues have been examined by Corney (1982) in a report on two small-scale surveys, one carried out in a group practice team and the other in a health centre team. Both teams contained general practitioners, district nurses, health visitors, and an attached social worker. However, only the group practice team also contained a CPN. The members of both teams were given a hypothetical list of social problems that their patients or clients could present, and asked who would be the most appropriate professional to deal with each. The researchers found marked disagreement in the answers from different disciplines, with most of the participants seeing themselves as dealing with a wider range of problems than their fellow team members thought. There was also a great deal of overlap in the roles of different disciplines, this being most marked between the health visitor and the social worker. The report also indicates that there could be overlap between the social worker and the CPN. In the health centre team without a CPN member the attached social worker received referrals of those people with relatively minor mental health problems (including depression and anxiety) and interpersonal problems. Two other reports of social worker attachment to primary care teams without attached CPNs report similar findings (Winny and Rushton, 1981; Phelan *et al.*, 1984). Corney suggests in her report that these referrals would probably have gone to the CPN had there been one.

The general practitioners in the studies felt that the CPN attachment had reduced both the number of referrals to psychiatric services and the amount of psychotropic medication they prescribed. Interestingly, it had not reduced their workload, but it had helped by enabling the sharing of the emotional burden of caring for people with psychiatric illnesses, and had offered a better service to those registered with the practice. It was considered a positive benefit that the attached workers would be seen as part of the health centre staff by patients/clients. The potential problems and conflicts that could arise from the overlapping of roles were obviated by regular team meetings where patients/clients could be discussed and any disagreements voiced. Corney concludes by suggesting, as others have done, that one of the major advantages of such attachments is that the different professionals involved get to know each other personally.

In the CPN's role of secondary prevention the primary health care team is therefore very much a part of the CPN system. As we indicated earlier, in the future general practitioners may also take on a much more active role with people having long-term psychiatric illness as ex-hospital patients move into accommodation in the local community. For both the long-term and short-term client groups good links between primary health care teams, CPNs and other mental health workers will be essential. We advocate that such links with all those working in primary care settings should be actively developed by CPN services, but that the partnership with in-patient psychiatric services discussed earlier should at the same time remain a positive commitment.

Finally, it may appear that we are advocating that one CPN should take on this wide range of work. In fact we suggest that a CPN service as a whole should over time move in these directions, with different members of the team taking on different elements of the task. No single CPN could or should be expected to carry responsibility for all such developments.

Social services

Since the implementation of the Seebohm report on the organisation of social service departments in 1971 there have no longer been specialist mental welfare officers, and social workers previously employed to work with mentally ill people have, along with other specialised workers, been absorbed into generic teams. As already outlined in Chapter 3, this development contributed to the growth of CPN services in the 1970s. It also continues to affect the work of CPNs today. For example, large generalist social work teams covering a patch can result in a CPN liaising with a number of different social workers, particularly if the client has not been allocated to an individual social worker's caseload but is being dealt with by the duty team. In addition, Hunter (1980) suggests that, perhaps because of their lack of specialised mental health training and their own perception of a lack of skills, some social workers in local authority area offices may see people with mental health problems as their least preferred client group. However, social workers are one of the main groups of professionals working in the community, and Hunter has argued that in the future social workers and CPNs are likely to be the two largest professional groups in contact with clients having mental ill-health in the community. It is therefore particularly important that the two disciplines are able to work well together.

Donnelly (1977) has suggested that social workers and CPNs must accept some overlapping of their respective roles, and has urged collaboration through face-to-face contact and joint work rather than competition. Once again the need for the members of different disciplines to know each other personally is recognised as essential to good working relationships. But what are the roles that the two professions share? An attempt to list the roles of social workers in relation to clients with mental ill-health has been made by a social worker (Hudson, 1976):

- *Statutory duties* – in particular under the Mental Health Act, and in taking children into care.
- *Helping clients to obtain material resources* – accommodation, benefits, home helps, meals-on-wheels, mobility aids and so on; sometimes this may entail acting as an advocate with, say, the housing department.
- *Assessment* – especially social history and home circumstances.
- *"Support for treatment"* – helping the client to make use of what is offered, and supporting relatives.
- *Psychosocial treatment* – counselling, often focusing on a particular current problem.
- *Community work* – working with groups or organisations.

Many CPNs would see themselves as taking on from time to time all but the first of these functions. Assessment, support for treatment, and often counselling are now generally considered to be amongst the skills of a CPN. In many districts CPNs will also liaise with social security offices, or request home helps or meals-on-wheels for their clients. It is often not appropriate to introduce another worker into a family to coordinate such services. In addition, some CPNs, like social workers, work with groups in the community. There is, therefore, some overlapping of roles. There are also other potential sources of conflict. At times CPNs have felt that social workers have pulled out once the former have become involved with a new client or family, leaving the CPN feeling unsupported and at a loss about how to proceed. By contrast, social workers could sometimes feel that they get little help from CPNs when there is a crisis that appears to require compulsory admission under the Mental Health Act.

The social worker's statutory responsibilities under the 1983 Mental Health Act are, of course, unchanged by the emergence of CPN services or by the Seebohm reorganisation. However the 1983 Act stipulates that only those social workers who are deemed to have appropriate qualifications and experience can be appointed as Approved Social Workers (ASWs), and only ASWs can exercise the powers conferred by the Mental Health Act. The Act also contains further implications for social work practice not contained in the 1959 Act. For example, it requires that the ASW personally interviews the patient, investigates the least restrictive treatment setting possible (by having a detailed knowledge of local provision), and considers the possibility of preventing compulsory admission by crisis intervention, informal admission, or support to the family (Gostin, 1983). Further, if compulsory admission is necessary the ASW should remain involved with the client and family to pave the way for a return to the community. Although some of these responsibilities cannot be shared with other disciplines, it is clear that there are considerable opportunities for working partnerships to be developed between ASWs, CPNs and other mental health professionals.

Where such working together does not happen there is potential for interprofessional rivalry and feelings within both disciplines of being threatened by the other professional group. We have already mentioned the need for personal contact and greater understanding of each other's roles in order to prevent this. Two examples (among many others) of how this could be done come to mind. First, all students on a particular post-registration RMN course spend one day per week in a social services team during their eight-week CPN placement. This not only gives the student nurse a good understanding of the role, functions and work pressures of social workers, but it also brings together individual CPNs and social workers through the need to plan the students' placements. Second, lunch-time meetings have been held every two or three months between hospital-based social workers and CPNs to get to know each other and discuss their work. These meetings, instigated by field workers rather than managers, have gradually drawn in other staff from the area offices, and are now seen as a valuable forum.

It is also extremely beneficial for joint clinical work to be established, whether it be joint visits to a particular family, or perhaps the joint running of a community support group. Sharing and joint working are needed at all levels of the respective organisations, so that both the delivery of care, and the planning, development and management of new community services for mentally ill people may benefit from a joint perspective which sees community psychiatric nursing and social work as complementary rather than competing.

Voluntary organisations

Earlier in this chapter we pointed out that the provision of community mental health services is shared by health authorities, local authorities and voluntary organisations. Many voluntary organisations have an important part to play: in *services* set up specifically for people with mental illness, such as sheltered workshops, day centres, drop-in centres, or after-care hostels; for *disadvantaged groups* who may or may not have mental ill-health, such as hostels for homeless people, advice centres, or street agencies for unemployed and rootless young people; or in *disseminating information* among both the public and professionals about schizophrenia for example, and providing support to families. Again, it is very important that CPNs find out which agencies operate in their area, what services they offer, how to refer clients to them, and whether the agencies know of the existence of the CPN service and how to contact it.

Voluntary organisations have the potential to be more flexible in the planning and delivery of services than a large organisation like the NHS can be. However, they pay for that flexibility by often having an insecure financial situation, in that they rely on various funding bodies (sometimes health or local authorities) to make grants to them each year. They do not see themselves as setting up services that are alternatives to those provided by the statutory organisations, but rather as establishing complementary services that are enhanced by remaining independent.

They are generally managed by a voluntary management group made up of interested lay people, representatives from local statutory services, local businesses, and so on. The larger organisations may delegate to a number of subcommittees that take on particular aspects of the work. As CPNs become more known to the staff and management groups of voluntary agencies with whom they have links they may be asked to join these management groups. This can be extremely valuable work as it gives the CPN the opportunity to bring his or her knowledge of the locality, and of potential clients of the agency, to bear on the agency's discussions about the current service and future developments. It can also help the CPN to gain a better understanding of the work of the organisation. However, it is important that the CPN is not seen by the voluntary organisation as representing the official views of the health authority, but that his or her contribution is made as a local fieldworker. It will certainly be very helpful for the CPNs doing such work to discuss it regularly with their nurse managers, so that they may be able to clarify "which hat they are wearing".

Accountability and the Law

The development of the systematic use of nursing assessments and care plans, developments in nursing education, and the growth of research have all contributed to the claim for nursing to be established as a profession in its own right. If we accept nursing as a profession, then "every professional person is responsible for his or her professional acts" (Baly, 1983, p. 229). In other words nurses are expected to be and remain safe practitioners, and to keep up to date, and they can be held accountable for this. This is particularly important where nurses work mainly on their own as CPNs do.

The legal adviser to the CPNA has pointed out that CPNs could be especially vulnerable in certain areas of the law, not only because they often work alone, but also because they are more likely to deal with people who may act irrationally at times (Carr, Butterworth and Hodges, 1980; Carr, 1984). In relation to this, Carr emphasises the need for health districts to have policies in particular on the carriage, storage and administration of drugs by CPNs, and on carrying passengers in their cars. In addition, he points out that the nature of CPNs' work may mean that they are more vulnerable in the future to having a civil action brought against them by a client or family for, say, negligence or breach of confidentiality. Several professional organisations now provide indemnity insurance for their members to cover such eventualities. At present CPNs are also occasionally required to give evidence at inquests or in child care cases. For all these reasons it is very important that CPNs communicate well with relevant colleagues about their work with a client, and record care plans and ongoing notes accurately and carefully.

Data Collection

Almost all CPN services collect a certain amount of data on clients and CPN activity on a weekly or monthly basis. This is often seen to be an arduous and, in some cases, largely irrelevant activity by the CPNs involved. Sometimes they may understandably wonder what, if anything, happens to their figures once they are handed in. Nevertheless, at several different points in this book we have argued that it is very helpful to the provision of a good service that CPNs record information about the locality in which they work and the people who are referred to them, while always bearing in mind the need for confidentiality, and remembering that information is given to them as trusted professionals by their clients. Some might answer that they often know a great deal about their clients based on long experience and their comprehensive nursing assessments, but they may be unable to present this information to others or use it in the planning of their own services, unless it is collected in a systematic way. One senior nurse in community psychiatric nursing has put it forcefully (Coulter, 1983, p. 7):

> The funding of the NHS will, no doubt, continue to decline in real terms and each service will have to fight even harder to maintain its share of funds. I would argue that those services which can clearly demonstrate what they are doing and that this is being done in the most economical way, will be the ones to develop and expand whilst the others will remain static or indeed may even decline.

A number of projects have attempted to collect such information systematically; for example, Coulter's study demonstrated the potential use of microcomputers in carrying out a community psychiatric nursing audit, and McKendrick (1984a) has for some years been collecting data on all those clients on his own caseload, and information collected daily about his work patterns.

Bloomsbury CPN service has been collecting information on all new clients referred to the service, and on CPN monthly activity since 1983 (see Brooker (1984) for a full discussion on setting this up). The client variables are almost all based on information that would usually be collected in the course of the CPN's initial assessment. The variable list and the categories for each variable were drawn up and amended in a series of meetings of all the CPNs involved. As a result, by the time the data collection started there was general commitment to the project. The list of variables has since been revised, again with full discussions in the team, and the main ones now are:

- age
- sex
- marital status
- ethnic background (collected because the service thought that people from ethnic minority groups may not be referred and therefore would not be receiving a service)
- the client's, referrer's and CPN's view of the problem
- problem duration
- occupation
- type of accommodation
- living arrangements
- main source of income
- referrer
- medication on referral and discharge
- previous psychiatric history
- diagnosis (if any)
- main CPN intervention
- number of home visits.

(The current list of variables and their categories are given in Appendix 3.)

Many of these variables are the same as those devised by McKendrick. It can be seen that almost all of this information is usually readily available to CPNs in the course of their assessments.

The monthly activity data refer mainly to a breakdown of how the CPNs allocate their time and information about their workloads. These include the amount of time spent in clinical and nonclinical activities (for example, liaison meetings, teaching sessions), and on numbers of referrals, discharges, and current caseloads.

The data are put on computer in a form that maintains confidentiality and does not identify individuals. In addition, the database must be registered with the Registrar of the 1984 Data Protection Act. This Act is based on principles which require that data are fairly and lawfully obtained and processed, accurate and kept up to date, and used only for the specific purposes given on registration (Wright, 1985).

Generally, anyone who is the subject of such a data file, who has information about themselves recorded in this way will, i they apply, be entitled to check their entry. However, the Secretary of State will determine whether records dealing with mental or physical health will be exempt from this "subject access".

Once the data are computerised and analysed this exercise gives us some very useful general information about the range of clients referred to the service and their overall characteristics, and how the service operates. This information, as we mentioned in Chapter 3, can be used in planning. In the future comparisons could be made between CPN services which cover districts with different characteristics or work in different ways. The data collected would then contain certain standard variables and also some variables that reflect what are seen to be the particular characteristics of the area concerned. Currently such comparisons are not possible. Indeed, McKendrick (1984a) refers to an earlier study in which he found little agreement among CPN services on what information was thought relevant to the measurement of CPN activity. Both McKendrick and Coulter (1983) argue for an agreed information package that would be used by all services. Indeed some progress has been made along this path by several regional health authority working parties looking at just such a minimum standardised CPN database. However, the success of such ventures crucially depends on the energies and investment put in by those collecting the basic data, in this case the CPNs. It is important that they are able to see the value in taking on such work.

There is, of course, a relationship between the systematic collection of such information and the need for a CPN service to have a strategy for its future direction and development. Such a strategy requires regular reviewing to assess to what extent its aims have been met. Data collection provides one mechanism by which this can be done.

The Political Systems of the CPN

There are two main ways in which the wider political system has a bearing on the work and role of the CPN. The first is in the context of the nursing profession as a whole, the second in the politics of the provision of health and community care of which CPN services are a part.

The statutory structure of nursing

In 1983, after a transitional period with shadow authorities, a new statutory structure for nursing, based on the 1979 Nurses, Midwives and Health Visitors Act, took over from the large number of previously existing bodies. These five new bodies, made up of elected and appointed members, are the United Kingdom Central Council for Nursing, Midwifery and Health Visiting (UKCC), and the National Boards for England, Wales, Northern Ireland and Scotland.

The main function of the UKCC is to "establish and improve standards of training and professional conduct for nurses, midwives and health visitors' (1979 Nurses, Midwives and Health Visitors Act, quoted by Hall, 1985, p. 17). It is therefore responsible for:

- establishing standards of training (in conjunction with the national boards)
- determining statutory criteria for entry to training
- determining criteria for registration
- establishing and maintaining the professional register
- establishing standards of conduct for the profession.

To these ends the council has, over the past few years, published a series of consultation papers on various subjects, and has attempted to seek the views of, and make its work widely known to, members of the profession. It has also issued the Code of Professional Conduct which aims to increase awareness amongst nurses of what can reasonably be expected of a registered nurse in terms of accountability and responsibility.

The national boards have a complementary function to that of the UKCC. They are primarily responsible for approving nurse training courses – both pre-registration and post-registration – and the clinical placements used by courses. Education officers cover specific geographical areas and take on an advisory and inspecting role for institutions proposing to set up new courses or continue established ones. The boards also draw up syllabuses for educational courses, for example the ENB course 811 (Nursing of the Mentally Ill in the Community) which is an update of the previous 810. The English National Board has also proposed a new educational strategy based on common core elements of nursing education prior to students moving to specific areas, which incorporates supernumerary status for nurse learners in the early part of their training.

Representative organisations

A number of different organisations represent the interests of nurses, including trade unions and professional organisations, and also organisations concerned with specific nursing groups. The Community Psychiatric Nurses Association (CPNA) is such an association for CPNs. This body has its roots in two separate developments in the mid 1970s, one in the north-west of England, and the other in the southern part of the country (Timms, 1985). Quite unknown to each other two groups of CPNs came together to encourage professional development (at a time when CPNs were still fairly thin on the ground) and to act as a pressure group for the working conditions of CPNs. When the two groups discovered each other in 1976 they amalgamated and formed a national organisation with, at that time, 120 members. Since then there has been a huge increase in the membership, and the association has grown considerably in status and influence.

The annual general meeting of the CPNA has, for a number of years, been linked to a training conference which has become increasingly popular and draws CPN members and non-members from all over the United Kingdom. Recently more and more of the sessions at the conference have been conducted by CPNs, suggesting that through such a forum CPNs have welcomed the opportunity to inform each other about their work. The association is organised into regions with regional coordinators who organise local meetings, discussions, training workshops, etc. The CPNA has also extended its aims to examining clinical practice, education, and the developing role of the CPN. It has submitted evidence on behalf of its CPN members to the Social Services Committee on community care, and to the DHSS Community Nursing Review. The association's bimonthly journal is circulated to all members and is a useful forum for discussion and sharing of information.

There are other organisations which attract CPN membership; for example the Royal College of Nursing has now established a Community Psychiatric Nursing Forum as one of its specialist groupings, and a number of meetings have been held in different parts of the country. In addition the Psychiatric Nurses Association (PNA) has a membership drawn from nurses working in the whole range of psychiatric services, including CPNs. The CPNA and PNA have already had some joint conferences, and there is a joint committee made up of representatives of all three organisations which has also organised conferences. Clearly all such organisations, focusing as they do on psychiatric nursing, and in some instances on community psychiatric nursing, could play an important part in the future development of this professional group, and in representing community psychiatric nursing to the outside world.

Should community nursing be political?

It has become something of a catch-phrase to say that "nurses should be political" without there necessarily being a very clear or agreed definition of what this means in practice. The winner of the 1985 Bard nursing award has pointed out that "to many nurses, getting political is synonymous with banner-waving and strike action" (Smith, 1985), but she argues that the work of nurses in the community must inevitably bring home to them the relationship between socio-environmental factors and health, and the implications of this relationship for nurses taking action should not be ignored. She outlines a number of different activities in which nurses could become involved including: increasing awareness of issues through reading the local and national press; joining and becoming actively involved in a professional organisation or pressure group; becoming involved in local or national politics.

The 1985 primary health care conference also took the question of a political role as one of its main themes, demonstrating that it is seen as an important factor in the future directions to be taken by community nursing. Although it is not possible to go into the surrounding ideas in any depth here, it may be helpful to highlight some of the key issues for CPNs.

Two interlinked themes arise in discussions of the nurse's political role – advocacy and professionalism. We discussed advocacy and the debate surrounding it in Chapter 5, so we shall not consider it further here, apart from a look at the relationship between advocacy, professionalism and the political role of nurses.

It has been suggested that the attempts within nursing to establish itself as a profession and to define professionalism means that nurses will move further away from their patients and clients and become an élite modelled on the profession of medicine. Salvage (1985) has put forward a case against the moves towards professionalism, arguing that it means keeping knowledge within the profession, rather than sharing it with clients, families and the general public; and that it reinforces the status quo, rather than questioning and pushing for change. If this were the case then the professional role of nurses would clearly be incompatible with the role of advocate. However, Salvage does not argue that professionalism must inevitably result in this. Speaking at the primary health care conference on this subject she has been quoted as urging nurses to "... redefine professionalism as a creed of excellence based on an alliance with the people who use our services" (*Nursing Times*, 1985, p. 6). In other words, it is important for nursing to see one of its main aims as being the fostering of a close working relationship between those who provide the service and those who use it. Smith (1985) also urges this and makes the telling point that providers of a service can also be its consumers.

What would this close working relationship mean in practice? As far as CPNs are concerned there are, we suggest, two main implications. The first is the need for CPN services to be in touch with user groups and to be working with them and with staff in other mental health services, to find out what kind of community mental health service is required, and then helping to bring that about. Second, the discussion brings us back to the issue of advocacy. We know that many people who have had a psychiatric problem may feel lacking in confidence, and for this or some other reason are unable to express their needs and wishes to others. CPNs working with them may take on such a role, and if they pursue it may indeed find themselves challenging the decisions of government departments or local authority organisations, such as DHSS offices or housing departments, on behalf of their clients. The appropriateness of such work has been raised by others (Mangen and Griffith, 1982, p. 159):

> To what degree should the nurse as a "community" care agent involve herself in the wider political context shaping the social situation of her patients, many of whom may be seriously deprived? It is open to doubt that, in the present situation, many community psychiatric nurses will want ... to assume an advocacy role in matters such as housing, welfare rights, unemployment and retraining. Yet these could be the issues most problematic for some

of her patients. . . . The advocacy role could be a distinct function of community psychiatric nursing in the future.

In addition the evidence is accumulating that both mental and physical health are greatly affected by social, environmental, financial and work-related factors (discussed in part in Chapter 2). Those CPNs and other community nurses who work in inner-city areas in particular will be very aware of the effects of national and local political decisions on the lives of their clients. If we begin to challenge and question these we are indeed taking on a political role.

Summary

In this chapter we have covered a range of different aspects of CPNs' work concerned with their relationships with members of their own team, their nurse managers, colleagues in mental health services and those outside. We have also considered organisations and developments at national level which create some of the context within which CPNs work. On a day-to-day basis many CPNs may think little about these issues, but nevertheless they can have a great impact on what happens in CPN services and the pattern of future developments.

References

Baly, M. (1983) Professions and professionalism, in Clark, J. and Henderson, J. (eds), *Community Health*. Churchill Livingstone, Edinburgh.

Brook, P. and Cooper, B. (1975) Community mental health care: primary team and specialist services. *Journal of the Royal College of General Practitioners*, **25**, 93–110.

Brooker, C. (1984) Some problems associated with the measurement of community psychiatric nurse intervention. *Journal of Advanced Nursing*, **9**, 165–74.

Brooker, C. (1985) Community mental health services in Italy: the implications for community psychiatric nurses in the United Kingdom. *Community Psychiatric Nursing Journal*, **5(3)**, 11–18.

Carr, P. J., Butterworth, C. A. and Hodges, B. E. (1980) *Community Psychiatric Nursing*. Churchill Livingstone, Edinburgh.

Carr, P. (1984) Legal and ethical perspectives in the nursing care of the mentally ill. *Community Psychiatric Nursing Journal*, **4(5)**, 14–18.

Corney, R. (1982) Team-work is a mixture of professional personalities. *General Practitioner*, **29**, 54–5.

Corser, C. and Ryce, S. W. (1977) Community mental health care: a model based on the primary care team. *British Medical Journal*, **2**, 936–8.

Coulter, D. (1983) The CPN, the microcomputer, and the nursing audit. *Community Psychiatric Nursing Journal*, 3(5), 4–9.

Donnelly, G. (1977) Relationships: the social worker and the psychiatric community nurse. *Nursing Mirror*, **22 September,** 39–40.

Fingret, A. (1985) Stress at work. *The Practitioner*, **June, 229,** 547–55.

Firth, H. W. B. (1984) Sources of good staff support. *Nursing Times*, Occasional Paper, **80(18),** 60–2.

Goldberg, D. (1985) *Mental health policies in Lancashire*, presented at Joint DHSS/ Royal College of Psychiatrists conference on community care.

Gostin, L. (1983) *A Practical Guide to Mental Health Law*. MIND, London.

Hancock, C. (1984) How to beat burnout. *Senior Nurse*, **1(34),** 18–21.

Hall, Dame C. (1985) The way forward. *Senior Nurse*, **2(1),** 16–18.

Hicks, C. (1984) An aide to better community care? *Nursing Times*, **11 January,** 8–10.

Hudson, B. (1976) The community psychiatric nurse and the social worker. *Nursing Times (Community Care Supplement)* **27 May,** xviii–xii.

Hunter, P. (1980) Social work and community psychiatric nursing – a review. *International Journal of Nursing Studies*, **17,** 131–9.

Manchester, J. (1985) The clinical factor. *Senior Nurse*, **3(2),** 51–2.

Mangen, S. P. and Griffith, J. H. (1982) Community psychiatric nursing services in Britain: the need for policy and planning, *International Journal of Nursing Studies*, **19(3),** 157–66.

McCarthy, P. (1985) Burnout in psychiatric nursing. *Journal of Advanced Nursing*, **10,** 305–10.

McKendrick, D. (1984a) Community psychiatric nursing data: a home computer system in operation. *Community Psychiatric Nursing Journal*, **4(2),** 5–11.

McKendrick, D. (1984b) CPN: cog or lever. *Nursing Times*, **80(7),** 36–8.

Nursing Times (1985) Speakers debate nurse's role as the patient's advocate. **81(42),** 6.

Menzies, I. (1960) A case study in the functioning of social systems as a defence against anxiety. *Human Relations*, **13(2).**

Phelan, L., Otlet, A. Smith, P. and Hanstead, P. (1984) Just what the doctor ordered. *Social Work Today*, **17 December,** 18–19.

Robertson, H. and Scott, D. J. (1985) Community psychiatric nursing: a survey of patients and problems. *Journal of the Royal College of General Practitioners*, **35,** 130–2.

Salvage, J. (1985) *The Politics of Nursing*. Heinemann, London.

Sharpe, D. (1982) GP's views of community psychiatric nurses. *Nursing Times* **6 October,** 1664–6.

Skidmore, D. and Friend, W. (1984). Muddling through. *Nursing Times, Community Outlook*, **9 May,** 179–81.

Smith, S. (1985) Political animals. *Nursing Times, Community Outlook*, **December,** 4–10.

Timms, C. (1985) The early days of the Community Psychiatric Nurses Association. *Community Psychiatric Nursing Journal*, **5(5),** 15–16.

Tough, H., Kingerlee, P. and Elliott, P. (1980) Surgery attached psychogeriatric nurses: an evaluation of psychiatric nurses in the primary care team. *Journal of the Royal College of General Practitioners*, **30,** 85–9.

White, E. (1986) Factors which influence general practitioners to refer to community psychiatric nurses, in Brooking, J. (ed.) *Readings in Psychiatric Nursing Research*. John Wiley, Chichester.

Winny, J. and Rushton, A. (1981) Social work in a health centre. *Health and Social Services Journal*, **6 March,** 257–9.

Wright, G. (1985) Micro-column. *Community Psychiatric Nursing Journal*, **5(2),** 38–9.

7
The Future Role of the CPN

The preceding six chapters have been guided by two important principles. The first is that CPNs and their clients are part of and relate to various systems. For the client this can mean being part of a family or relating to the complex organisation of a psychiatric hospital. The CPN's systems can be just as complicated: at any one time in the working week a CPN can be a CPN team member, part of the primary health care team, and a contributor to the in-patient care team discussing a client's impending discharge home.

Second is the belief that a CPN's role is ultimately the responsibility of each CPN. Thus we have not said what CPNs should do in any given situation. Instead the factors that affect CPN practice have been outlined, leaving the ball firmly in the reader's court.

This final chapter examines some important issues for CPNs that have not been covered in detail elsewhere – the CPN and nurse education, CPN specialism versus CPN genericism, and the CPN and the future.

The CPN and Education

The year 1985 heralded many developments in the field of nurse education. It was, in fact, the year of the "nurse education blueprint". First on the scene was the Royal College of Nursing which produced an extremely well-researched document on the future of nurse education, the now-famous Judge Report (RCN, 1985). Next the English National Board produced their consultative document also on the restructuring of nurse education (ENB, 1985). Finally, the United Kingdom Central Council (UKCC) provided nursing with some informative background material in discussion papers called *Project 2000* (UKCC, 1985).

Many factors prompted the RCN, ENB and UKCC to look at basic nurse education in this depth, and we have chosen to discuss only those that seem most relevant to CPNs. These are the ambiguity of the student's status (employee versus student); the changing emphasis in health care from cure to prevention; the implementation of a new curriculum based on a nursing model; the declining number of students applying for basic RMN training and indeed the projected decrease in numbers of places available; and finally the logistical problems of providing a meaningful educational experience for students in the community.

This last problem has arisen because of the new RMN training syllabus (1982) which has as one of its main aims to increase the experience gained by RMN learners in the community. It is possible, using the new syllabus, to map out a course of training for an RMN learner that over 3 years involves only 9 months placement in in-patient settings. Two factors are essential for such a training course. First, the District Health Authority (DHA) must have a comprehensive range of community-based service provision for the learner's placements, and second, the CPN service must have enough committed personnel to provide a meaningful educational experience for the learner. This is at a time when the educational demands on CPNs come not just from RMN students, but from district nurses, community occupational therapists and medical students, at an ever-increasing rate.

Skidmore and Friend (1984b) have looked at the demand that the change in the basic RMN syllabus will place on CPNs, and questioned the value for students of their current attachment to CPNs. In their study, 63% of students interviewed after placement with CPNs held a negative view of the CPN. Skidmore and Friend state (p. 259): "Students on the whole, left the placements with an inaccurate or vague picture of what community psychiatric nurses actually do, or what teams are capable of achieving." Their research also looked at the student placement from the CPN's point of view; 80% of CPNs reopened old and "safe" cases for the student's benefit because they perceived a threat from the student (in terms of harming the CPN–client relationship) if he or she were to accompany them on visits to active cases. This is a most unsatisfactory state of affairs for both student and CPN.

We shall now turn to the actual proposals put forward by the RCN, ENB and UKCC and consider the possible implications of these proposals for CPNs.

The RCN's proposals

The Judge Report firmly backs the principle of full-time student status for the nurse learner based in a centre of full-time further education. The RCN envisages a three-year course, leading to a diploma in nursing studies which would then be recorded on a single professional register. The first year would be a common foundation course with an emphasis on health promotion. The second year would involve three practical placements, in the community, nursing adults in hospitals and finally in a variety of settings related to mental health. In the final year of the course, the student would specialise in one of six areas, including mental illness, and the RCN advocates that the specialty followed should be recorded on a single register. On completion of the diploma, the nurse would then need to work in the appropriate clinical area for six to 12 months with an experienced practitioner, in a module of staff development. Finally the nurse would then have the option of undertaking an advanced diploma in a clinical specialty or progressing to pursue degree studies.

Unfortunately, the implications of these proposals for CPNs are not clear. The RCN's document concentrates entirely on revisions to basic nurse education; thus the issue concerning mandatory postbasic training for CPNs is sidestepped. The modules proposed for "mental illness" specialisation in the third year are ambiguous and no direct mention is made of community-based experience, although one module is entitled "The mentally ill in non-institutional settings". Furthermore, there appears to be some tension between the emphasis on "health promotion" in the first year of training and the subsequent use of the phrase "mental illness" in the third year options. Clearly the RCN's proposals require much further discussion in relation to the future training needs of CPNs.

The ENB's proposals

The ENB's proposals are not unlike the RCN's but they do differ in several respects. First, while all students would share a common core in the first year of training, after this they would separate out, aiming for registration on the existing parts of the register. In the third year students would become salaried again and experience would be almost entirely gained in clinical areas. Appendix 4 of the ENB's document states: "There will be a continuing need to provide advanced preparation for mental nurses to practise in specific settings (for example, community psychiatric nursing . . .)" (Section 5 (ii) p. 27). This presumably would become an option under the advanced diploma schemes outlined as one-year postbasic courses after initial registration. These courses, the document stresses, must from the beginning be based in colleges of further education. Again, it is not clear whether postbasic courses for CPNs should be mandatory. We shall return to this issue.

The UKCC's proposals

The UKCC's deliberations began in 1983 under the auspices of their educational policy advisory group. In 1985 this committee produced six project papers that addressed issues such as the future of the enrolled nurse, "student" status for nurse learners, whether nurses should be "generalists" or "specialists", and the future health care needs of the population by the year 2000. The UKCC states that in comparison to the ENB's work "Project 2000 has a much wider remit and is looking at how professional preparation should be developed to meet future health care needs. It is not taking the present legislation as a constraint. . . .". (p. 5). Perhaps, therefore, we can expect very radical proposals from the UKCC, but at this stage it would be impossible to predict their meaning for CPNs.

Training for CPNs: mandatory or not?

The proportion of all CPNs holding the postbasic qualification in 1980 was 24.2%. By 1985 this had decreased to 22.4%, and in that year only 618 CPNs completed a postregistration course in community psychiatric nursing (Joint Board of Clinical Nursing Studies course number 800/810, ENB cc number 810 or the Scottish or Northern Ireland equivalents). This means that since the CPNA survey of 1980 there has been an increase of 303 in the numbers of CPNs holding the certificate.

Further data from the national boards for nursing, midwifery and health visiting show that since CPN training started in

England in 1974, 1095 certificates have been awarded to nurses completing JBCNS course number 800/810, and ENB cc number 810 (a separation is unavailable for those completing the mental handicap option in JBCNS course number 800). In Scotland, CPN training began in 1980 and to date 84 certificates have been awarded (including those of the Scottish National Board successor.) Northern Ireland's course began in 1982 and has now awarded 42 certificates. There is no course in Wales at present. Therefore, a total 1220 certificates have been awarded, but only 50% of these nurses are practising clinically at present. It is likely that many of the remaining 50% have been promoted to service managers. Butterworth (1985) identified this as the only promotion possibility for the CPN.

At present in England 11 centres offer ENB cc number 810 and 811 with a total of 246 places available a year. This number is slightly reduced due to the fact that at five of the 11 centres there is an unidentifiable number of places on ENB cc number 805 (the mental handicap option). A new centre has been approved recently in Warwick to run a 20-place short course, ENB cc number 992, for those CPNs who have been practising for three years or longer.

Table 7.1 CENTRES APPROVED FOR ENB CC NUMBERS 810/805 OR 811

Centre	Course	Number of places
North-east London Polytechnic	810	24
Birmingham Polytechnic	810	15
Manchester Polytechnic	810/805	70
Newcastle	810	10
Bristol Polytechnic	810	12/15
Barking	810	10
Sheffield Polytechnic	810/805	25
Portsmouth	810/805	12
West London Institute	810/805	30
Northampton	810	15
North-east Surrey	811	20
	Total	246

These are the facts, then, so what are the arguments for mandatory CPN training? In 1982, the CPNA and the RCN issued a joint statement entitled "Mandatory training for CPNs – the way forward". The argument for mandatory training in this document is based on the view that basic psychiatric nurse training does not prepare a nurse for community-oriented work and does not provide specialist skills training. However, this document predated the publication of the new 1982 RMN syllabus, and it has been argued that once the new products of this course emerge training for CPNs will no longer be necessary (Brooking, 1985). Nevertheless, there still remain the current difficulties. More and more CPNs are being appointed to posts with no previous community experience, and many more will be before significant numbers of the "new RMN syllabus product" emerge in the 1990s. Thus the CPNA continues to advocate mandatory training. In their response to the Short Report on Community Care (CPNA, 1985), the CPNA stated:

> We repeat that the CPNA commitment to mandatory training, the increasing numbers of CPNs and the pressing need for a clinical career structure will have important cost implications. Further training centres and teachers are required as it is clear that training establishments ... are unable to keep pace with the increasing number of new appointments.

Whatever one's point of view on mandatory training one issue seems clear. In Chapter 3 we saw that the huge projected increases in CPN personnel over the next decade or so are related to closing large psychiatric hospitals. In the main, this will mean that CPN service priorities should be directed at providing support structures for long-term institutionalised patients. Many different skills will be required to effect such strategies, skills which are rare at present. How many CPNs can say they are skilled in teaching activities of daily living to chronically handicapped people living in the community for the first time in 20 years? How many CPNs are adept at the public relations required to prepare a community for a new residential project? These undoubtedly will be some of the new skills all psychiatric nurses, not just CPNs, will require.

The CPN and Clinical Specialism

CPN specialism refers to a CPN working exclusively with one client group; in contrast, a generic CPN intervenes with clients of all ages and with every sort of problem. Table 3.3 in Chapter 3 shows that nationally in 1985 793 CPNs (approximately 35% of all CPNs) specialised exclusively in any one area. Perhaps then it seems redundant to discuss whether or not CPN specialism is a good idea! However, we know that the numbers of CPNs specialising with the elderly vary dramatically throughout England, from 33% of the workforce in the Wessex region to only 10% in the Trent region (CPNA, 1985b). This suggests that the degree to which specialisation is thought to be important differs greatly throughout the country, so let us look at both sides of the argument.

Carr, Butterworth and Hodges (1980) discussed whether a CPN should be a generalist or a specialist and linked this with education. They predicted that most CPNs would be generic to begin with but stated that (p. 179): "... eventually they will specialise e.g. in psychogeriatrics or with children etc. Perhaps the typical CPN of the future will have three trainings; basic, community psychiatric, plus one specialism." One way to put this into practice would be a skills-based modular course for CPNs, a course not unlike the one Carr and his colleagues currently run at Manchester Polytechnic.

Some people, such as Mangen and Griffith (1982, p. 158), argue that CPNs should not take on a generic role because it reduces their effectiveness. Generalism, they also argue, could ensnare CPNs in one particular role which might be well below their actual potential. Mangen and Griffith believe that if generalism is to become the way forward then mental health services would be better off encouraging ward-based nurses to work in the community as a part-time commitment—a belief we think is unrealistic.

Mangen and Griffith then go on to argue that if a greater proportion of CPNs are to become specialists, there would be better use of resources if they were more involved with patients still in hospital. In any event, they say services should be centred on out-patient departments or health centres and less emphasis should be placed on domiciliary services. This seems a strange argument to come from one of the authors of the controlled trial at Springfield Hospital, a study which showed that clients preferred CPNs to out-patient appointments, one of the reasons being a preference for being seen in their own homes (Paykel and Griffith, 1983)!

Skidmore and Friend's (1984a) research into the role of the

CPN specialist found that specialists are seen to be élitist, escapist and arrogant. This was concluded after observing over 1000 visits from a random nationally-selected CPN sample. This research serves some timely warnings – for example, there are dangers that CPN services will develop into a collection of mutually exclusive specialists and that clients who do not fit neatly into a specialty will be neglected: "Many potential clients were overlooked because they did not fit into the rigid borders of the specialism and clients were dealt with via the limited intervention strategy of the specialism, particularly by the behaviourists" (Skidmore and Friend, 1984a, p. 203).

Interestingly enough Skidmore and Friend point out that many CPNs specialising in behaviour therapy had been unsuccessful applicants for the ENB cc number 650 course in behavioural psychotherapy. These CPNs also often felt directionless when newly appointed as a CPN. On the positive side, however, their research did show that there were no significant differences in patient outcome between specialists and generalists. Furthermore, specialists were found to be more confident in their role than their generalist colleagues.

There has been little research into the work of CPNs who specialise. Brooker and Brown (1986) followed up all graduates of ENB cc number 650 in behavioural psychotherapy. This survey showed that 8.2% of qualified nurse therapists called themselves CPNs, while 25.5% (the largest proportion) based their work in community psychiatric nursing departments but did not actually call themselves CPNs. However, the most important difference between nurse therapists and CPNs is how they view the importance of clinical supervision; 82% of the nurse therapists stated that no-one supervised their day-to-day clinical work. This finding is related to the course's aim which is to produce "an autonomous therapist". The study concludes (p. 192): "The survey's findings suggest that nurse therapists' closest professional allies are CPNs. The way this relationship develops in the future should be an area of immediate concern for both groups. One obvious possibility is an examination of the salient elements of both . . . training programmes".

Kennedy (1986) surveyed CPNs specialising with clients with alcohol problems, a study aimed at establishing the training needs of CPNs working in community alcohol teams (CATs). He found that CPNs working in CATs are undertrained and, in particular, that they need to develop behavioural and psychotherapeutic skills beyond the level reached during basic nurse training. Kennedy suggests that, as CPNs make up 70% of the personnel working in CATs, these training needs must be rectified immediately.

To conclude this debate on CPN specialism we would like to reiterate our concern about hospital closure policies and their impact on future CPN training needs. The 1985 CPNA survey indicated that in the UK there were only 42 CPNs specialising in rehabilitation. Furthermore, there are few suitable postbasic training courses for CPNs that relate to the needs of institutionalised people (see Brooker and Beard, 1985).

We believe that some CPNs should specialise and that they should then work in teams where the majority of colleagues are generic CPNs. We also believe that when CPNs do specialise they must be appropriately trained for the role. It is the responsibility of individual CPNs and their managers to determine local priorities for specialist training. As large hospitals close, courses will be required to develop specialist skills for rehabilitation work. A serious commitment is required from seconding DHAs to send a CPN on a full-time course, such as ENB cc number 811, as course fees are expensive and the CPN is lost from the service for the 9 months' duration of the course. There are at present around 2000 untrained CPNs working in the United Kingdom and nationally about 250 places annually on ENB cc number 810/811 (and its equivalents). It would therefore take eight years to train all current CPNs, if no new CPNs were appointed during this period. If the argument for mandatory training is based on the need for CPNs to develop specialist clinical skills, ENB cc number 810/11 will not always provide a relevant educational experience. There are many local part-time day-release clinical skills courses and these may also be appropriate, especially for CPNs who already have a lengthy experience in the community.

The CPN and the Future

Research

This book has consciously incorporated relevant research findings into the text. We would like now to discuss the future direction in which we think CPN research should go.

In Chapter 3 we deplored the "topdown" approach to planning the number of CPNs required in each DHA, which was usually related to the concept of CPN manpower planning targets and population ratios – for example, the now infamous one CPN per 10 000 DHA population. We strongly believe that CPN workforce requirements should emanate from the "bottom-up" from individual CPN service managers. This means that the task of CPN managers is to make some estimate of future local need, and this requires research into the following factors:

(1) *The characteristics of the DHA, including age structure, rural versus urban mix, and the incidence of mental health problems.* Some of this information will certainly be available from census data, and local CPN data collection should provide the rest. There is also information about social deprivation available for each DHA in England (Rice, Irving and Davies, 1984).

(2) *The individual DHA's strategic/operational proposals for the continuing development of comprehensive district mental health services.* Certainly CPN managers should be involved in any such planning discussions particularly where hospital closure is an issue (see the CPNA's policy statement on closure of large psychiatric hospitals – CPNA, 1985a).

(3) *The style and organisation of each individual DHA's existing CPN provision.* For example, CPN services that are hospital-based and consultant-attached would seem to have a finite capacity for expansion, whereas services that are more community oriented will have more inherent flexibility in the way that they develop.

(4) *The range and extent of local requirements for specialist CPN services. These may include services for drugs and alcohol, rehabilitation and those for elderly people.*

Future staffing levels for individual CPN services should never be divorced from the overall strategic plan for mental health services in any one district; CPN service managers should be producing operational proposals, based on researched local assessment of need, but running parallel with wider district plans.

Consumerism

Another important subject for research is consumer satisfaction – how satisfied our clients are with the care we give them. This is to be taken particularly seriously by CPN services given the importance now paid to it by new general management arrangements and the recent report from the Community Nursing Review (DHSS, 1986).

There has been some research in this area: Paykel and Griffith (1983) looked at consumer satisfaction, Simmons (1984) examined consumerism in relation to family carers, and we are aware that a major piece of research by Pollock into consumer satisfaction is soon to be published. In general, however, we know little about the type of service our clients want.

At an organisational level, it is felt (largely intuitively) that clients require a CPN service that is local, accessible and flexibly delivered – in other words, available outside normal office hours. However, an evaluation of a London counselling service (James, 1985) has shown that such a service can be used very infrequently. This study concludes that local and accessible services also have a very high community profile. Consequently, the stigma attached to being seen using it by neighbours is so great that in fact potential clients are discouraged from visiting.

It has to be accepted that CPN research into consumer satisfaction presents formidable methodological problems (Lebow, 1982). But these problems are worth overcoming because the client has a unique view of the treatment process and vitally important ideas about the quality of that service. We as CPNs must take heed of the client's view in a much more systematic way.

Performance indicators

Apart from consumer satisfaction there are a number of other basic indices, or performance indicators, that could be developed to allow comparison of CPN services nationally. Nearly all CPN services collect some basic data, both about clients referred to the service and CPN caseload activity. We would like to see the development of basic standardised performance indicators so that individual Districts and Regional Health Authorities could compare CPN service performance.

Future research

The final point we would like to make about future CPN research is the necessity of repeating the 1980 and 1985 CPNA surveys in 1990. Over the next five years there will be great change in all aspects of CPN team work and organisation, and it will be vital to map these changes and keep pace with the hectic developments that are inevitable.

Implications of the Community Nursing Review (1986)

The Report of the Community Nursing Review (or Cumberlege Report) was published in early 1986. Its terms of reference were to "study the nursing services provided outside hospital by health authorities" and to report on how such resources might be used more effectively.

The report stated that while the general public's confidence in community nurses was high, a chain of weakness had developed, which included problems such as:

● Individual and community needs not being systematically identified.
● Routine collection of data which have little value.
● Underutilisation of professional skills and duplication of effort by primary care team members, leading to lack of coordination.

The review team made several recommendations aimed at overcoming these difficulties, the major focus of which was the creation of neighbour nursing services (NNS), a team which would integrate the work of district nurses, health visitors and school nurses, for an identifiable neighbourhood of perhaps 10 000–25 000 people. The major implication for CPNs at this stage would be that CPN teams should ensure through their service manager that their work was fully coordinated with the NNS. It remains unclear what national impact the Cumberlege Report will have, not just on CPNs, but on all community nurses, as its recommendations have yet to be implemented by the government.

What will happen to the CPN?

In 1954, the first out-patient psychiatric nurse left the ward at Warlingham Park Hospital to visit a client at home. In 1986, 40 community mental health workers will be operating from five community mental health centres in the Exeter Health Authority. The contrast in style of care delivery is great indeed. The concept of community care, initiated by Tooth and Brook's (1961) erroneous statistical predictions and set in motion by Enoch Powell's *Hospital Plan* (Ministry of Health, 1962), seems to have come of age.

During this era, CPNs have in a sense been sitting on the sidelines waiting for everybody else to catch them up. Now that they have, what does the future hold? The most obvious response is perhaps a change in name. CPNs, in Exeter at least, have metamorphosed into "community mental health workers" (CMHW). As CMHWs they will be working in multidisciplinary teams consisting of social workers, psychologists and one consultant psychiatrist. The community mental health centre base will provide a walk-in, easy-access service to a population of approximately 40 000–50 000 people. The skills required of CMHWs in these teams have been described by Pope (1985) as skills in assessment, counselling, family therapy, group work, problem-solving and evaluation. The community mental health centre provides a crisis service, an assessment centre and a resource for mental health workers, and has a responsibility to ensure that people suffering from chronic mental illness receive a service. The change in name from CPN to CMHW has been of fundamental philosophical importance. The rationale is that "mental health" can only be effectively promoted in the appropriate social context – the community – whereas psychiatric illness was always previously treated in a psychiatric hospital. We can foresee that in the next five to ten years the name CPN will gradually be phased out and alternatives such as the CMHW will replace it. This was brought home to us when we were trying to decide what to call this book!

The other change of emphasis that we can confidently predict, given the plans of Exeter and other DHAs, is that CPNs will become increasingly involved with multidisciplinary teams based in the community. At present the tendency is for generic CPN teams to be attached individually to psychiatrists and GPs but to share a common base. This can be very useful for sharing problems and gaining peer supervision. Specialist CPNs at present are more likely to be found working, say, in multidisciplinary teams for the elderly or in community alcohol teams. However, as hospitals reduce in size and eventually close, territory formerly claimed exclusively by the CPN will have to be shared with other professional colleagues, in particular, psychologists, psychiatrists and social workers. This will require a radical reorganisation of working practices, and there may well be heated debate and problems over clinical responsibility, referral patterns and role overlap, particularly in relation to CPNs and social workers. MIND (1983), in their blueprint for the future of mental health services, predict these difficulties and suggest that a possible solution is the widening of the current CPN training course to train a new group of professionals entitled "community mental health workers".

Another area of concern for the future is what will become of staff nurses, state enrolled nurses, and nursing assistants in future community mental health services? At present these grades make up 14% of the total national CPN workforce or one in seven, a sizeable proportion.

Skidmore and Friend (1984c) examined the role of the SEN in community psychiatric nursing in some detail, relating it to the SEN's counterpart, the RMN. The SEN group spent longer in client contact, were more patient-centred and appeared more confident than their RMN colleagues. The researchers say that at a time when there is a move to phase out the SEN in nursing altogether, we should reconsider the latter's role in community psychiatric nursing. Melia (1984), in an appraisal of a scheme for elderly people in East Dorset, found that care assistants (or nursing assistants) provided a service, under the direction of a trained RMN, judged by relatives to be infinitely preferable to hospitalisation.

There is, then, a very real role for staff nurses, SENs and nursing assistants in community nursing; furthermore, as hospitals close there is an obligation to provide employment for nurses in those grades, some perhaps as peripatetic workers in clients' homes, others in community residential schemes. One thing is certain – the problem will not be a lack of jobs for psychiatric nurses of these grades, but a lack of nurses to fill the posts.

Summary

In this chapter we have looked at desirable research trends, the pronouncements of the Community Nursing Review, and predicted trends in community psychiatric nursing over the next few years.

However, we do not want to leave the reader feeling that the future of community psychiatric nursing is in complete flux. Change in the health service and in our professional roles as CPNs usually leads to development and growth. This has certainly been the case for CPNs over the last three decades, and hopefully will continue to be so.

In 1961, Goffman wrote: "If all the mental hospitals in a given region were emptied and closed down today, tomorrow relatives, police, and judges would raise a clamour for new ones; and these true clients of the mental hospital would demand an institution to satisfy their needs." It is our sincere hope that as hospitals close Goffman will be proved wrong by CPNs. For it is largely in the hands of CPNs that the future shape of mental health service lies.

References

Bendall, E. (1977) The Future of British Nurse Education, *Journal of Advanced Nursing*, **2**, 171–81.

Brooker, C. and Brown, M. (1986) National follow up survey of practising nurse therapists, in Brooking, J. *Readings in Psychiatric Nursing Research*. J. Wiley and Sons, Chichester.

Brooker, C. and Beard, P. (1985) Psychiatric nursing – quo vadis? *Bulletin of the British Journal of Psychiatrists*, **9**(4), 70–2.

Brooking, J. (1985) Advanced psychiatric nursing education in Britain. *Journal of Advanced Nursing*, **10**, 455–68.

Butterworth, A. (1985) Mandatory training for community psychiatric nursing. *CPNA Conference Review Supplement*, 3–5.

Carr, P. J., Butterworth, A. and Hedges, B. E. (1980) *Community Psychiatric Nursing*, Churchill Livingstone, Edinburgh.

Community Psychiatric Nursing Association (1985a) Policy statement on the closure of large psychiatric hospitals. *Community Psychiatric Nursing Journal*, **5**(5), 44–5.

Community Psychiatric Nursing Association (1985b) *The 1985 National CPNA Survey Update*, CPNA Publications, Leeds.

Community Psychiatric Nursing Association (1985c) CPNA response to the social services committee report. *Community Psychiatric Nursing Journal*, **5**(3), 46–8.

DHSS (1986) *Neighbourhood nursing – a focus for care. Report of the Community Nursing Review*. HMSO, London.

English National Board (1985) *Professional Education/Training Courses* (a consultative document). ENB, London.

Goffman, E. (1961) *Asylums*, Penguin, Harmondsworth.

James, C. (1985) *An evaluation of a drop in counselling service*, Unpublished thesis, South Bank Polytechnic.

Kennedy, J. (1986). A national survey of community alcohol teams. *Nursing Times* – to be published.

Lebow, J. (1982) Consumer satisfaction with mental health treatment. *Psychological Bulletin*, **91**(2), 244–59.

Mangen, S. and Griffith, J. (1982) Community psychiatric nursing services in Britain: the need for policy and planning. *International Journal of Nursing Studies*, **19** (3), 159–65.

Melia, A. (1984) *An evaluation of the East Dorset home care project*. Brunel University, unpublished.

MIND (1983) *A Common Concern*. MIND Publications, London.

Ministry of Health (1962) *The Hospital Plan*. HMSO, London.

Paykel, E. S. and Griffith, J. (1983) *Community Psychiatric Nursing for Neurotic Patients*. Royal College of Nursing, London.

Pope, B. (1985) Psychiatry in transition – implications for psychiatric nursing. *Community Psychiatric Nursing Journal*, **5**(4), 7–13.

Rice, P., Irving, D. and Davies, G. (1984) *Information about District Health Authorities in England from the 1981 Census*. King's Fund Centre, London.

Royal College of Nursing (1985) *The Education of Nurses: a New Dispensation*. Royal College of Nursing, London.

The Short Report (1985) *Community Care: with Special Reference to Adult Mentally Ill and Mentally Handicapped People*. House of Commons Paper **13(1) Vol. 1,** HMSO, London.

Simmons, S. (1984) *Family burden – what does it mean to the carers?* Unpublished MSc thesis, Surrey University.

Skidmore, D. and Friend, W. (1984a) Specialism or escapism? *Nursing Times (Community Outlook)*, **13,** 203–5.

Skidmore, D. and Friend, W. (1984b) Student rethink needed. *Nursing Times (Community Outlook)*, **11 July,** 257–61.

Skidmore, D. and Friend, W. (1984c) CPNs need enrolled nurses. *Nursing Times (Community Outlook)*, **8 August,** 299–301.

Tooth, G. C. and Brook, E. M. (1961) Trends in the mental health population and their effect on future planning. *Lancet*, **1 April,** 710–13.

United Kingdom Central Council (1985) *Project 2000* (Project Papers 1–6). The Educational Policy Advisory Committee, London.

Voluntary Organisations and Agencies

Age Concern – England
Bernard Sunley House, 60 Pitcairn Road, Mitcham,
Surrey CR4 3LL. 01 640 5431

Age Concern – Northern Ireland
6 Lower Crescent,
Belfast BT7 1NR. 0232 245729

Age Concern – Scotland
33 Castle Street,
Edinburgh 031 225 5000

Age Concern – Wales
1 Park Grove,
Cardiff CF1 3BJ. 0222 371821

Al-Anon Family Groups
(help for relatives and friends of problem drinkers)
61 Great Dover Street,
London SE1 4YF. 01 403 0888

Alcohol Concern
(national agency on alcohol problems and referrals to local
services)
305 Grays Inn Road,
London WC1 8QS. 01 833 3471

Alcoholics Anonymous
General Service Office, PO Box 514,
11 Redcliffe Gardens,
London SW10 9BQ. 01 352 9779

Alzheimer's Disease Society
3rd Floor, Bank Building, Fulham Broadway,
London SW6 1EP. 01 381 3177

Anorexic Aid
(voluntary self-help groups)
The Priory Centre, 11 Priory Road, High Wycombe,
Buckinghamshire (send SAE for local contact)

Association of Carers
(self-help groups for carers)
First Floor, 21/23 New Road,
Chatham
Kent ME4 4QJ. 0634 813981/2

Association for Postnatal Illness
(network of phone and postal volunteers)
Institute of Obstetrics and Gynaecology,
Queen Charlotte's Hospital, Goldhawk Road,
London W6

Child Poverty Action Group
(national body campaigning on poverty in families)
1 Macklin Street, Drury Lane,
London WC2B 5NH. 01 242 3225/9149

Cruse: National Organisation for the Widowed and their
Children
(counselling service with local branches)
Cruse House, 126 Sheen Road, Richmond,
Surrey TW9 1UR. 01 940 4818/9047

Families Anonymous UK
(for families and friends of those with drug problems)
88 Caledonian Road,
London N1 9DN. 01 278 8805

Gay Switchboard
(information and help for gay men and women)
BM Switchboard,
London WC1N 3XX. 01 837 7324

Gingerbread
(self-help groups for one-parent families)
35 Wellington Street,
London WC2E 7BN. 01 240 0953

Health Education Council
(information and leaflets on health subjects)
78 New Oxford Street,
London WC1A 1AH. 01 637 1881

Mencap
(advice, help and information for mentally handicapped people
and their families)
123 Golden Lane,
London EC1Y 0RT. 01 253 9433

Mental Aftercare Association
(residential accommodation, help and support for ex-psychiatric
patients)
Eagle House, 110 Jermyn Street,
London SW1Y 6HB. 01 839 5953

MIND
(National Association for Mental Health)
22 Harley Street,
London W1N 2ED. 01 637 0741

National Council for Carers and their Elderly Dependents
(information and advice for those caring for dependent relatives)
29 Chilworth Mews,
London W2 3RG. 01 724 7776

National Marriage Guidance Council
(national coordinator of local councils)
Herbert Gray College, Little Church Street, Rugby,
Warwickshire CV21 3AP. 0788 73241

National Schizophrenia Fellowship
(help, advice and support for relatives)
78/79 Victoria Road, Surbiton,
Surrey KT6 4NS. 01 390 3651

Philadelphia Association
(accommodation and refuge on psychotherapeutic model for
people in mental distress)
14 Peto Place,
London NW1 4DT. 01 486 9012

Psychiatric Rehabilitation Association
(day and residential care, and support for ex-psychiatric patients)
The Groupwork Centre, 21a Kingsland High Street,
London E8 2JS. 01 254 9753

Rape Crisis Centre
(counselling, medical and legal help for women who have been
raped or assaulted)
PO Box 69,
London WC1X 9NJ.
01 278 3956 (office hours); 01 837 1600 (24 hours)

Release
(24-hour advice on drug use, drug problems, criminal law)
c/o 347 Upper Street,
London N1 0PD. 01 289 1123

Richmond Fellowship
(counselling, halfway houses and group homes for those with
mental ill-health)
8 Addison Road,
London W14 8DL. 01 603 6373

The Samaritans
181 branches in UK and Eire
Telephone numbers in local directories under S

Tranx
(advice and support for those taking tranquillisers; information
on setting up self-help groups)
17 Peel Road, Harrow,
Middlesex HA3 7QX. 01 427 2065

Turning Point
(rehabilitation for people with drug or alcohol problems – day
centres and residential houses)
CAP House, 4th Floor, 9–12 Long Lane,
London EC1A 9HA. 01 606 3947/9

Women's Therapy Centre
(counselling and psychotherapy for women
and their families, also workshops and groups)
6 Manor Gardens,
London N7 6LA. 01 263 6200

A Strategy for the CPN Service

Introduction

The Social Services Select Committee Report on Community Care (1985) endorses the Health Advisory Service (HAS) view that: "The CPN is probably the most important single professional in the process of moving care of mental illness into the community" (para 192); and goes on to say: "CPNs are in the community to provide expertise in psychiatric care equivalent to the best nursing care available in hospitals" (para 193).

We do not, as yet, have a generally agreed definition of what constitutes equivalent good nursing care in the community, and the future direction of services. In this document a strategy is put forward that goes some way to addressing this.

The CPN Service

The Community Psychiatric Nursing Service (CPNS) has grown fairly rapidly over the past few years so that there are now 17 charge-nurses divided into three teams, each with its own leader.

The team leader role is clinically oriented, with a strong commitment to providing supervision and leadership to team members, in addition to some management responsibility. In the light of the comments of the Select Committee and the growth in the service, it is now particularly important that future developments and use of resources are coordinated with the overall strategy for mental health services, and that there is a consistency in the direction taken by the CPNS as a whole.

Aims of the CPN Service

The key elements of the strategy are as follows:

The CPN service aims to provide an accessible local service, and offers care for people with a wide range of mental health problems living in the community. There is a team responsibility for providing a generic service (within which are areas of special expertise) that will continue to adapt and respond flexibly to the changing mental health needs of the population, in particular with the planned closure of X Hospital and the development of a self-sufficient district service. It is, perhaps, essential that the development of small specialised components of the service is not detrimental to the generic team, since it is thought that over-specialising in a CPN service does not allow for the flexibility and adaptability that are needed by a varied population.

It is recognised that it is important to remain genuinely responsive to what is needed by the local community, rather than what professionals feel able to, or wish to, provide. This will entail maintaining a balance within the service between meeting the needs of both those with long-term mental illness and short-term mental health problems.

The CPN service will therefore aim to be:

- local – as far as possible based in the community it serves
- accessible to clients, referrers and other enquiries
- for clients and families with a wide range of problems, including those who need long-term care
- flexible in the delivery of care, both by providing a range of interventions, and in using a variety of settings and times.

Operational Implications of these Aims

The intention is to continue to develop community bases for CPNs, mainly in health centres and health clinics. However, problems arise due to limited office space, and access to interview or group rooms. Where it is appropriate to a particular development in the service CPNs may also be based in other agencies, for example, a social services department. They may also work elsewhere on a sessional basis, for example running a group in a community centre. A CPN based in a clinic or health centre offers a geographical service as well as liaising with the primary health care workers in the clinic.

In order to develop accessibility a leaflet has recently been printed and circulated. It will be important for circulation to be maintained through already existing distribution networks.

Links with Community Services

The CPN service sees the provision of community mental health care as a joint responsibility shared by the mental health services, primary care, social services, and voluntary agencies. The greater part of psychiatric disorder is treated by general practitioners. However, many general practitioners work single-handedly and are likely to have less access to the back-up psychiatric services. It is therefore intended to improve links with general practitioners so that referrals both to the CPN service and to the psychiatric services as a whole can be facilitated, and the local population receive a more coordinated service. It is envisaged that these links will be established by each CPN contacting a small number of general practitioners in his or her area on a regular basis; this process has already begun.

The CPNS plans to continue developing closer links with other nurses working in the community – that is district nurses, health visitors, geriatric visitors and school nurses etc. Where these nurses are not based in the same places as CPNs some regular meetings are already taking place between CPNs and other community nursing staff, and these will be further developed.

It is not the aim of the CPN service to become totally primary health care-oriented, however, since some residents do not have a general practitioner and will have to gain access to the service in other ways. Therefore development and maintenance of links with hostels, day centres, and voluntary agencies dealing with homeless and rootless people will be continued, by regular meetings with staff, involvement in management committees (where appropriate) etc.

Links with In-patient Services

It is also important to maintain a close working relationship with the in-patient areas, by taking an active part in planning for discharge and rehabilitation programmes, thereby promoting an integrated service. The CPN should be seen as a member of the ward team, which would necessitate regular contact (for example, fortnightly) with ward staff. Where CPNs are members of the ward team this could lead to sharing of nursing care (where appropriate) and direct involvement in community-oriented treatment programmes.

The ward team should also ensure that any CPNs are informed when their clients are being discussed in ward rounds so that they can attend.

Referral System

The referral system will remain as open as possible; telephone referrals (with a back-up letter or referral form) are welcomed. If the person is not referred by his/her general practitioner, the latter will generally be notified of the referral (unless the client does not wish this to be done). If the client is not registered with a general practitioner the CPN will encourage and help him or her to do so. First contact with the person referred will, whenever possible, be made quickly. (The CPN service does not at present provide an emergency service of "duty" system; the need for such a service requires investigation.) On occasion, it has been extremely helpful to involve the referrer in the first visit.

This and other types of joint work may be developed further.

Services for Elderly Mentally Ill People

The mental health unit operational plan proposes small multi-disciplinary teams caring for elderly mentally ill people in the community, of which at least one member would be a CPN. It will therefore be part of the CPN service strategy for some of the CPN input for this age-group to be made as a member of these teams, although the nurses involved would continue to have links with the CPN service. It is also envisaged that all generic CPNs would continue to carry a number of old people on their caseloads in addition to the specialist services.

Rehabilitation

This is already a part of the CPN's role, but will become more so as community care progresses. CPNs could become involved with hospital residents prior to discharge, concentrating particularly on aspects of the transition that may cause difficulties or stress. The support would then be continued once the individual is discharged, if he or she moves into unstaffed accommodation. It may become necessary to develop different ways of working with some clients, for example concentrating longer periods of time on daily living skills, or taking part in social clubs and activities. This may entail working closely with other disciplines, such as community occupational therapists, and might involve regular contact and a rapid, intensive response in times of crisis.

Such an area requires a different pattern of work and possibly additional training. There may be a need for particular CPNs in this field to act as "resource people" for both CPN colleagues and others.

Other Client Groups

The CPN service has also recognised that there are groups of potential clients who may need special provision since they may have no access to the service through normal channels; these include ethnic minority groups, and homeless people. It is envisaged that particular CPNs should develop interest and knowledge in these areas; the CPN service recognises the need for nurses with special understanding of different ethnic groups, and this could be met by employing a wider ethnic mix of staff, through possibly some change in recruitment policy within the health authority.

Community-based Multidisciplinary Teams

It is also mental health unit policy to establish small community teams catering for a particular client group or area. These projects will contain nurses, some of whose work will overlap with the CPN service as a whole. It is therefore essential that there is a good flow of communication between the different services, and that although the special project nurses may not be members of the generic CPN service there is a well-established link, reflected in the nursing management structure.

The Work of Psychiatrists in the Community

As more people are treated in a community setting in the future there will be an increasing need for psychiatric input in people's homes, hostels and in health centres and clinics. The Health

Advisory Service suggests that one or more posts should be established of community psychiatrists who would be able to work closely with members of the CPN service, primary health care workers and hostels; CPNs strongly support this recommendation. Until recently CPNs have tended to be the main mental health personnel working in the community. However, this is already changing with the appointment of community occupational therapists and it is important that CPNs work closely with other professionals moving out of an institutional setting.

Staffing and Hours of Working

Currently CPNs generally work during office hours, Monday to Friday, with occasional evening work. However, as more psychiatric care is being provided in the community, it may become necessary for the CPN service to adopt a more flexible pattern of time allocation – for example, flexitime, regular evening shifts, and weekend work – and this would generally be focused on particular developments, and integrated with other out-of-hours provision.

The changing pattern of CPN work in the future, and the movement towards care in the community, may require employment of different grades of staff, just as different grades are currently employed in in-patient areas. Generally any staff nurses in the teams would be in training posts, and would carry less responsibility.

There may also be benefits in involving some volunteers in the service to provide clients with a kind of contact that professionals cannot give.

There should be opportunities for part-time working, and job-sharing without loss of promotion opportunities. Where a CPN works less than four days a week he or she would share a caseload with a colleague to provide continuity of care.

A health authority crèche would help to prevent the loss of staff who leave to have children.

Data Collection and Evaluation

The collection of data concerning those referred to the service, and CPN activity, will continue with regular reviews so that the

data collected are the most appropriate for monitoring the service
and planning new developments.

Data Coding Sheet

		Column number
1	Card Number 1	(1)
2	CPN Number	(2,3)
3	Case Number	(4,5,6)

4 Month of referral
   01 January
   02 February
   03 March
   04 April
   05 May
   06 June
   07 July
   08 August
   09 September
   10 October
   11 November
   12 December   (7,8)

5 Year of referral   (9,10)

6 Referral status
   1 New referral
   2 Transferred from another CPN
   3 Re-referral   (11)

7 Sex
   1 Male
   2 Female   (12)

8 Age (in years)   (13,14)

9 Marital status
   1 Single
   2 Married/cohabiting
   3 Widowed
   4 Separated/divorced   (15)

10 Ethnic background/identification
   1 Chinese
   2 Greek/Greek Cypriot
   3 Caribbean
   4 Indian subcontinent
   5 African
   6 Scottish
   7 Irish
   8 Middle-eastern
   9 Other   (16)

11 Referrer's view of main current problem
   01 Mood-related
   02 Abnormal experiences
   03 Drugs/alcohol
   04 Interpersonal relations
   05 Organic
   06 Financial/housing/employment
   07 Behavioural disturbance
   08 Recent loss or separation
   09 Anxiety
   10 Other
   11 None   (17,18)

12 Client's view of main current problem at first interview
   01 Mood-related
   02 Abnormal experiences
   03 Drugs/alcohol
   04 Interpersonal relations
   05 Organic
   06 Financial/housing/employment
   07 Behavioural disturbance
   08 Recent loss or separation
   09 Anxiety
   10 Other
   11 None   (19,20)

13 CPN's assessment of main current problem
      01 Mood-related
      02 Abnormal experienced
      03 Drugs/alcohol
      04 Interpersonal relations
      05 Organic
      06 Financial/housing/employment
      07 Behavioural disturbance
      08 Recent loss or separation
      09 Anxiety
      10 Other
      11 None   (21,22)

14 Problem duration
      1 Less than one month
      2 One month to six months
      3 Six months to two years
      4 More than two years   (23)

15 Employment status
      1 Regular
      2 Casual
      3 Unemployed
      4 Retired
      5 School/student
      6 Houseperson   (24)

16 If unemployed, how long (in months)?
      0 Not applicable
      1 Less than one month
      2 One month to six months
      3 Six months to two years
      4 More than two years   (25)

17 Main source of income
      1 Private
      2 Earnings
      3 State benefit/pension
      4 Dependent
      5 No income   (26)

18 Accommodation
  1 Owner-occupied
  2 Rented
  3 Hostel
  4 Bed and breakfast
  5 Sleeping rough
  6 Other   (27)

19 Referring agent
  01 General practitioner
  02 Social services
  03 Health visitor/geriatric visitor
  04 Psychiatrist
  05 District nurse
  06 Hostel
  07 Age Concern
  08 Probation Service
  09 Day centre
  10 Day hospital
  11 Ward staff
  12 West End Coordinated Voluntary Services
     (WECVS)
  13 Voluntary organisation (other)
  14 Self
  15 Other
  16 CPN   (28,29)

20 Is referring agent still involved?
  1 Yes
  2 No   (30)

21 Living arrangements
  1 Lives alone (including hostel)
  2 Lives with friend(s)
  3 Lives with spouse/cohabitee
  4 Lives with spouse and children
  5 Lives alone with children
  6 Lives with parents
  7 Other   (31)

22 Prescribed psychotropic medication, on referral
    1 Minor tranquillisers
    2 Major tranquillisers
    3 Antidepressants
    4 None
    5 Other   (32)

23 Prescribed psychotropic medication on discharge
    1 Minor tranquillisers
    2 Major tranquillisers
    3 Antidepressants
    4 None
    5 Other   (33)

24 Main intervention following assessment
    1 Drug supervision/administration
    2 Supportive/practical help/health education
    3 Counselling/psychotherapy
    4 Family therapy
    5 Behaviour therapy
    6 Referred on
    7 Other
    8 None
    9 Lost contact   (34)

25 Has client ever been seen by a psychiatrist?
    1 Yes
    2 No   (35)

26 If yes, how long ago was the last contact the
    client had with a psychiatrist (in months)?
    0 Not applicable
    1 Less than six months
    2 Six months to two years
    3 More than two years   (36)

27 Which of the following diagnostic categories most
aptly describe the formal psychiatric diagnosis given?
 0 Not applicable
 1 Affective disorder
 2 Schizophrenic disorder
 3 Personality disorder
 4 Dementing process/senile dementia
 5 Anxiety state
 6 Alcoholism/drug abuse
 7 Other
 8 Not known   (37)

28 Has the client ever been in a psychiatric hospital as a
patient?
 1 Yes
 2 No   (38)

29 If yes, how much time elapsed between last
discharge and CPN referral?
 0 Not applicable
 1 While in hospital
 2 Within six months
 3 Six months to two years
 4 More than two years   (39)

30 Did the client require psychiatric hospital
admission while on your caseload?
 1 Yes
 2 No   (40)

31 Total number of sessions with client   (41,42)

32 How many hours did you invest with this client
in total (including notes)?   (43,44)

CPN monthly activity

Column number

1 Card number 2 — (1)
2 CPN number — (2,3)
3 Number of sessions (in hours) in clients' home this month (round up sessions lasting less than one hour to one hour. Sessions lasting, say, two hours are recorded as two) — (4,5)
4 Number of sessions with clients at CPN's base this month (in hours) — (6,7)
5 Number of sessions with clients this month apart from those in the client's home or CPN's base (in hours) — (8,9)
6 Grand total of all client sessions this month (3,4 and 5 = 6) — (10,11)
7 Number of appointments missed by clients this month — (12,13)
8 Number of referrals — (14,15)
9 Number of discharges — (16,17)
10 Total number on caseload at end of month — (18,19)
11 Number deceased — (20,21)
12 Number lost contact — (22,23)
13 Number referred on — (24,25)
14 Number transferred to another CPN — (26,27)
15 Number no longer needing CPN service — (28,29)
16 Number of clients visited weekly or more often — (30,31)
17 Number visited between once weekly and once monthly — (32,33)
18 Number visited monthly or less often — (34,35)
19 Number of clients who have been on caseload for more than twelve months — (36,37)
20 Number of sessions (in hours) in CPN meetings — (38,39)
21 Number of sessions (in hours) liaison with hostels and voluntary agencies — (40,41)
22 Number of sessions (in hours) liaison with primary health care workers — (42,43)
23 Number of sessions liaison with other groups/agencies — (44,45)
24 Total number of liaison sessions (in hours) (= total of 21, 22, 23) — (46,47)

25 Number of sessions (in hours) in clinical
    supervision   (48,49)
26 Total number of teaching sessions given   (50,51)
27 Total number of teaching sessions attended   (52,53)
28 Month
    01 January
    02 February
    03 March
    04 April
    05 May
    06 June
    07 July
    08 August
    09 September
    10 October
    11 November
    12 December   (54,55)

Index